T0366035

# THE FIG
## THE MIRACLE FRUIT

## HEALTHY AND HEARTY EATING

HADI MIRRAFATI

A Special Message to All Athletes

Athletic performance is improved by high carbohydrate diets, not high protein diets. Protein supplements are expensive, unnecessary and even harmful for many people, especially athletes. Athletes need balanced sources of protein and carbohydrates, not concentrated protein. After eating any concentrated protein, like red meat, chicken, fish and milk products, the kidneys must cleanse the blood of protein wastes, such as ammonia, urea, and amino acid fragments. There is a predictable loss of calcium following the ingestion of concentrated protein. For hours after eating a piece of fish or meat, calcium pours out of your body with each urination. This is a well-known and reproducible phenomenon called "protein-induced hypercalcuria" and the calcium that is leaving the blood is being taken out of the body's vital storehouse of calcium—which are the bones. Strong and healthy bones are a very vital component of an athlete's body.

This calcium loss, year after year, drains calcium from the skeleton, resulting in thin, crumbly bones that fracture easily. This is known as osteoporosis. Osteoporosis is most severe in people who consume the most concentrated protein (red meat, chicken, fish, milk and milk products). Fruit and vegetable protein is less prone to cause calcium loss due to its slower absorption and less acidic nature.

Figs are the only fruits that athletes can depend on for protein, carbohydrates, vitamins, minerals and fiber, as well as enzymes. Athletes should definitely avoid fried foods, high-fat meals, lunchmeats, bacon, ham, chicken, fish, milkshakes, and any foods that are cooked in animal fats. Muscles need glycogen (a carbohydrate) for their fuel and carbohydrates give them the sustained energy they need for athletic activity. A basic complex-carbohydrate diet provides sustained, long-term energy. Proteins build tissue and fats provide lubrication and tissue support. Fiber allows good elimination. Female athletes need iron-rich foods, as their red blood cells may be broken down more rapidly. Figs do all of these as well as provide vitamins, minerals and salts.

Athletes: stay away from alcohol, cigarette smoking, coffee, black tea and cola beverages. Your best herb teas are green tea, ginseng tea, comfrey tea and white willow bark tea. For enhanced taste, use dried figs with your tea. Eat a few dried figs with a cup of green tea before you exercise, train or compete.

*To my sons*

*Kamran and Kamfar*

ISBN:   Softcover      978-1-4134-5463-5
        Hardcover      978-1-4134-5464-2
        EBook          979-8-3694-1979-3

To order additional copies of this book, contact:
Xlibris
844-714-8691
www.Xlibris.com
Orders@Xlibris.com

Print information available on the last page

Rev. date: 04/10/2024

# Contents

*Chapter One*

# THE
# MIRACLE FRUIT

There is something magical about trees that bear beautiful flowers and edible fruit. If you have a yard you can plant your favorite fruit trees and pick fresh fruit to eat when they are ripe. Fruit is filled with vitamins, minerals, fiber and enzymes, which humans need in daily life. You can preserve fruit in jams or in pies, cakes, pudding, rolls, baked breads, or freeze for later consumption. Your local produce mart will have ample fruit from which to choose. Among these, the miracle fruit, the fig, should be your first and daily choice.

## Fig Trees
Formally the Ficus carica of the Moraceae (mulberry) family, the fig is known as figue (French), feige (German), figo (Italian), and higo or brevo (Spanish). Figs are not technically fruits in the botanical sense; they are hundreds of

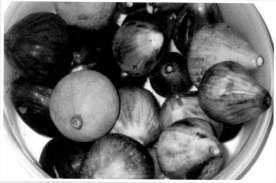

*Fresh Figs*

minuscule flowers encased in a fleshy balloon-like receptacles (syconium) that we term fruit. They are delicious, with great benefits. Figs contain fiber and minerals that are medically curative and dietetically delicious: **They can "clean inside" and help create a "youthful outside."**

The fig is a source of fiber. Fiber helps prevent constipation and colon cancer, and lowers cholesterol and thus the risk of heart disease. Three figs, dried or fresh, provide about 5 grams of fiber, 20 percent of Daily Values. That amount can go a long way. Figs are good for people who are overweight, another risk for heart disease. They stay in the stomach longer, helping people eat less. They are also very sweet, satisfying those cravings.

Figs can help prevent serious conditions that may affect you as you age. Figs can also satisfy your appetite and sweet tooth. You can prepare delicious, healthful snacks, desserts and main courses using the miracle fig.

## Origin and Distribution

The fig has been cultivated for centuries in warm, semi-arid climates, in western Asia and the Mediterranean area. Figs were part of the athlete's diet for the original Olympic games in ancient Greece. Even then, the fig was thought to be health-giving. Today we still call it **athlete's fruit** because of the terrific boost of energy it gives.

Figs grew from Afghanistan to southern Germany and the Canary Islands. Figs were introduced into England in the sixteenth century. By 1550 they were in Chinese gardens. European types were taken to China, Japan, India, South Africa, and Australia. The Spanish brought figs to Mexico, planted along such staple crops as grapevines and sugarcane in their new colonies. Thomas Jefferson brought three different varieties of fig home from France. The fig tree was common around Bahamian plantations. It became a familiar dooryard plant in the West Indies and at medium and low altitude in Central America and Northern South America. There are fair-sized plantations on mountain sides of Honduras, at low elevations on the Pacific side of Costa Rica, from Florida to northern South America, to Chile and Argentina where cooler zoned types are grown.

A century ago, figs were still a major crop in Florida, Virginia, and other southern states. Times and tastes changed but the fig has remained on the table and in the landscape. Turkish varieties are still a common sight in Florida, Georgia, Louisiana, Virginia, South Carolina, Tennessee and Mississippi. In California, figs were introduced when the San Diego Mission was established in 1769. In 1900, the wasp was introduced as the pollination agent to make commercial fig culture possible.

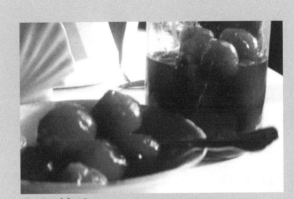

*Fig Breakfast Jam*

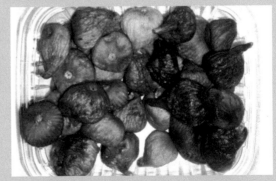

*Dried Calimyrna Figs*

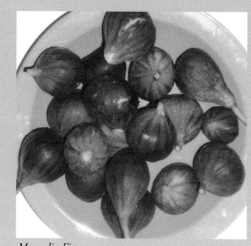
*Magnolia Figs*

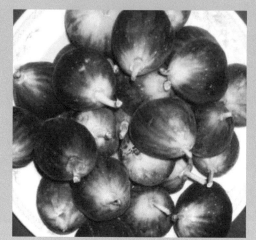
*Celeste or Honey Figs*

## VARIETIES

There are many cultivated varieties of figs. Some popular varieties suited to warm areas that do not require pollination are:

- Celeste (Blue Celeste, Honey Fig, Malta, Sugar, Violette)
  - o Pear-shaped, ribbed, with a short neck and slender stalk to ¾ inch long
  - o The eye (opening at apex) is closed
  - o The fruit is small to medium
  - o The skin is purplish-brown or bronze tinged with purple
  - o The pulp is whitish or pinkish amber
  - o Rich flavor, good quality and sweet, almost seedless
- Brown Turkey (Aubiquc, Noire, Negro Largo, San Piero)
  - o Broad-pyriform
  - o Usually without neck
  - o Medium to large
  - o Copper-colored
  - o Pulp is whitish shading to pink or light red with few seeds

- Brunswick (Magnolia)
  - o Leaves narrow-lobed
  - o Fruit is oblique-turbinate, mostly without neck
  - o Bronze or purplish-brown seedless fruit
  - o Pulp whitish near skin, shading to pink or amber, hollow in center
- Marseilles (Blanche, Italian Honey Fig, Lattarula, Lemon Fig, White Marseilles)
  - o Fruit round to oblate without neck
  - o Slender stalks to ¼ inch long
  - o Medium size, sweet
- Adriatic (Fragola, Strawberry Fig, Verdone, White Adriatic)
  - o Small to medium
  - o Skin greenish
  - o Flesh strawberry colored
- Genoa (White Genoa)
  - o Very faintly ribbed
  - o Neck thick and short or absent
  - o Distinctive flavor and good quality
  - o Medium size
  - o Skin downy, greenish-yellow to white

- o Flesh yellow-amber near skin, mostly amber tinged with red
- o Sweet, good for fresh or dried
- Purple Genoa (Black Genoa, Black Spanish)
  - o Oblong, broad at apex, narrow at base
  - o Large size
  - o Very dark-purple with thick blue bloom
  - o Pulp yellowish becoming reddish to red at the center
  - o Juicy and sweet with rich flavor
- Black Ischia (Blue Ischia)
  - o Pear shaped
  - o Short neck and short to medium stalk
  - o Dark purple-black except at the apex where it is lighter and greenish with many golden flecks
- Skin is fully coated with thin, dark blue bloom
  - o Eye open with red-violet scales
  - o Pulp is violet-red
  - o The tree is particularly ornamental and leaves are glossy
- Poona
  - o Bell shaped
  - o Medium size
  - o Thin skinned
  - o Light purple with red flesh
  - o Sweet with good flavor
- Black Mission (Bears Black, Franciscan)
  - o Fruits all over black-purple
  - o Elongated
  - o Flesh watermelon to pink
  - o Fairly good taste
  - o Easily dried at home
- Conadria
  - o Fruit pale green
  - o Medium size
  - o Flesh strawberry-red
  - o Mildly sweet
  - o Excellent dried

- Croisic (Cordelia, Gillette, St. John Fig)
  - o Only edible Capri fig
  - o Fruits pale yellow
  - o Small size
  - o Pulp nearly white

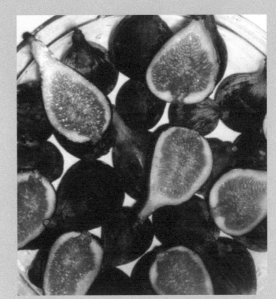

*Mission Figs*

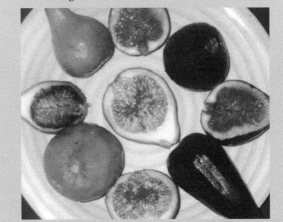

*Four Different Figs*

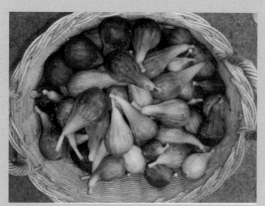

*Flanders Figs in a basket*

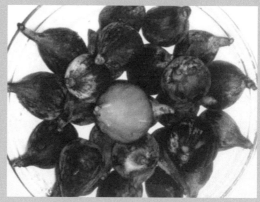

*Kadota Fig with a Plate a Missions*

- Desert King (Charlie, King Fig)
  - Large size
  - Skin is deep green, minutely spotted white
  - Pulp strawberry-red
  - Sweet
  - Delicious fresh or dried
- Excel
  - Large size
  - Skin is yellow
  - Flesh light amber
  - Fruits practically neck-less
  - Very sweet
- Flanders
  - Medium size
  - Long neck
  - Skin is brownish-yellow with violet stripes
  - Flesh amber
  - Strong, fine flavor
- Kadota (Dottato, Florentine, White Kadota)
  - Medium size
  - Skin yellowish-green
  - Flesh amber, tinged pink at center
  - Flavor rich

  - Resists souring
- Osborn's Prolific (Arachipel, Neveralla)
  - Medium to large
  - Skin is dark, reddish-brown
  - Flesh amber, often tinged pink
  - Very sweet
- Panachee (Stripped Tiger, Tiger)
  - Small to medium
  - Skin is greenish-yellow with dark green stripes
  - Flesh strawberry
  - Sweet
  - Best fresh
- Tena
  - Small size
  - Light green skin
  - Flesh amber
  - Fine flavor
  - Good fresh or dried
- Ventura
  - Large size
  - Green skin
  - Deep red flesh
  - Long neck

- o Excellent flavor
- o Good fresh or dried
- Vente (Green Ischia)
  - o Small size
  - o Greenish-yellow skin
  - o Flesh strawberry
  - o Excellent fresh or dried

Double your pleasure by growing fruit trees, not only for the fruit, but also for their ornamental and decorative value. If your yard is small, plant dwarf varieties or espalier, as a decorative screen to camouflage a sterile wall.

The first step is to select a suitable site. Most fruit trees need a sunny location and do best in well-drained soil. Select your plant according to your climate. Consider the plant's cold hardiness, which reflects the lowest temperature it can tolerate and survive during dormancy. Determine how your tree of choice is pollinated and whether or not it is self-fruitful. Help is available from your local nursery, and from university extension fruit specialists. Lastly, control and manage pest and disease

The roots of the fig tree are greedy, traveling far beyond the tree canopy; therefore, the fig tree is not for small places. The fine roots invade garden beds; however, they may be cut without loss to the tree. In areas with short, cool summers, espalier trees against a south-facing, light-colored wall take advantage of the reflected heat. In coastal climates, the fig tree grows in the warmest locations, against a sunny wall or in a heat trap. For container-grown plants, replace most of the soil in the tub every three years and shade the sides of the tub shaded to prevent over-heating in sunlight.

## Irrigation

Water young trees regularly until fully established. In dry western climate, water mature trees deeply at least every one or two weeks. Desert gardeners may have to water more frequently. Mulch the soil around the trees to conserve moisture. If a tree is not getting enough water, the leaves will turn yellow and drop. Dought-stressed trees will not produce fruit and are more susceptible to nematode damage.

## Pruning

Fig trees grow quite rapidly to a height between 15 and 30 feet. They are typically low branched and spreading. These fruiters are grown on their roots and can live for 100 years or more. Where hard freezes are common, the wood freezes back severely and the plant turns into a big shrub. In some colder areas, the plants will dry to the ground each winter, but will send up new shoots in spring. A fig can be trained as a formal or informal espalier. Most fig varieties produce two crops a year. The first is in early summer from wood formed the previous year. The second appears in late summer, born at the ends of new growth that formed while the first crop of figs was maturing. In colder climates only the second crop is produced, while in cool summer areas only the first crop ripens. A fig can take quite a bit of pruning, yet still bear an ample crop. It will also bear without pruning.

*Fruit Bearing Tree*

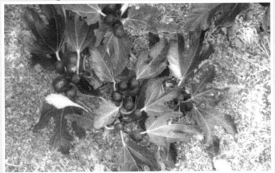

### Fertilization

Regular fertilizing of figs is usually necessary only for potted trees or when they are grown on sands. Excess nitrogen encourages rank growth at the expense of fruit production and the fruit often ripens improperly, if at all. Generally, fertilize fig trees if the branches grow less than a foot from the previous year. Apply about 1 pound of actual nitrogen divided into three or four applications beginning in late winter or early spring and ending in July.

### Frost Protection

In borderline climates, figs can be grown outdoors if given frost protection. Plant against a wall or structure which provides some heat by radiation. Grow as a bush and prune the trunk to near level at the end of the second year. Erect a frame over the plant, covering and surrounding it with heavy carpet in winter. Keep the roots as dry as possible during winter, raising a berm to exclude melting snow during thaws. In northern climates, the fig is best grown as a tub or pot plant that can be brought into a warm location in winter and taken out again in spring. Dormant buds are more susceptible to freezing than wood.

### Pests

Fig tree roots are a favorite food of gophers who can easily kill a large plant. One passive method of control is to plant the tree in a large aviary wire basket. Birds can cause a lot of damage to the fruit. Fig trees are prone to attack by nematodes, particularly in sandy soils, where they attack the roots, forming galls and stunting the trees. Driedfruit beetles can enter ripening fruit through the eye and cause damage by introducing fungi and knots. Asterolecanium attack the bark. Check with your nursery or local plant advisories to be sure your fig tree remains healthy and produces fresh food for your diet and health.

# Chapter Two

# THE ROLE OF FIGS IN YOUR HEALTH

Fresh figs are rich concentrates of a unique type of fiber within their tiny seeds. When you eat several fresh figs and drink fresh fruit juice or other favorite natural beverage, the seeds become liquefied and the fiber expands very gently so that the scrubbing action works comfortably and efficiently. Several figs "the night before" or early in the morning will boost inner cleansing so that the waste are actually scrubbed out of your body to improve the efficiency of your digestive system.

Dried figs are one of the best sources of natural fiber. Those delectable, succulent nuggets, rich in vitamins and minerals and delightful to the taste, are at least 35 percent higher in fiber than 40 percent bran flakes. Eating dried figs at mealtime as a quick snack assures adding a source of fiber and good nutrition, not just the fillers or empty calories found in many processed foods. Fine figs, fresh or dried, give you nine grams of good fiber. Figs are loaded with minerals and nutrients to help fend off heart disease, cancer, constipation, and even diabetes.

*Ready to Eat!*

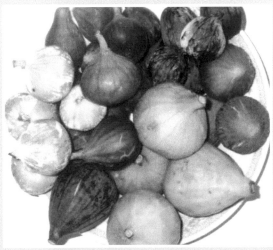

### Inner Cleansing

Figs help boost inner cleansing. Without fiber, food remains too long in the colon and causes bacteria and toxins to accumulate. The longer food is retained, the more water is absorbed leaving the waste material dry, hard and difficult to evacuate. Under normal conditions the colon produces mucus to protect the intestinal wall, which keeps the material moving at a regular and smooth pace. The colon loses its natural mucus when the water is absorbed and the feces attach themselves directly to the intestinal wall. This creates chronic diseases if not eliminated. Figs moisten the large intestine and balance acidic conditions that result from a diet of meat and refined food.

Bowel constipation over the years can back up into the venous, arterial, and lymphatic systems and enter every cell of the body. Old fecal matter will balloon the bowel and weaken it, allowing bacterial toxins to enter the blood stream. The toxins then poison the nerves surrounding the colon, ultimately affecting gall and other related tissue organs and systems.

The body retains high concentration of harmful bacteria. The toxins released by the decaying food move into the bloodstream, weakening the entire body. As the cecum becomes enlarged, the cecal valve can become incompetent and cause regurgitation into the small intestine, which allows dangerous poisons to be reabsorbed into the bloodstream. The enforcement glands cannot handle the toxin load. People could suffer for several days.

How much fiber do you need each day? Health authorities state that some 35 grams of fiber per day help protect against cancer as well as cholesterol overload. The larger you are, the more you need (a small person might require only about 25 grams daily). As you add more fiber to your diet, drink several glasses of good water a day. This helps compensate for any water loss due to the bulking properties of fiber. Large amounts of insoluble fiber increase bulk and draw water into the large intestine. The results are a larger, softer stool that exerts pressure on the colon walls and is eliminated more quickly indeed. The reduced pressure also helps prevent diverticulosis.

---

*A Word of Caution*:

If you have *Rosacea*, a condition that makes your nose and cheeks red and bumpy, you might want to avoid figs. Figs contain histamine, which causes flushing and can further irritate your skin.

Figs can also cause high blood pressure, headaches, and neck pain if you are taking a certain type of antidepressant called monoamine oxidase (MAO) inhibitor.

# Fiber Content (grams) In One 3.5 Ounce Serving

| | | | |
|---|---|---|---|
| Almond | 2.6 | Olives | 1.3 |
| Apples | 1.0 | Parsnips | 2.0 |
| Dried apricots | 3.8 | Peanuts | 2.4 |
| Artichokes | 2.4 | Pears | 1.4 |
| Avocados | 1.6 | Snow peas | 1.2 |
| Baked beans | 1.5 | Cooked pears | 2.0 |
| Blackberries | 4.1 | Raw peppers | 1.8 |
| Brazil nuts | 3.1 | Popcorn | 2.2 |
| Broccoli | 1.5 | Prunes | 2.2 |
| Brussel sprouts | 1.6 | Raspberries | 5.1 |
| Red cabbage | 1.0 | Rice bran | 11.5 |
| Carrots | 1.0 | Polish rice | 2.4 |
| Cashew nuts | 2.6 | Sunflower seed | 3.8 |
| Celery | 1.0 | Seaweed | 3.2 |
| Coconut meal | 4.0 | Kelp | 6.8 |
| Cranberries | 1.4 | Irish moss | 1.8 |
| Dates | 2.3 | Blueberries | 1.5 |
| **Fresh figs** | 2.1 | Sesame seeds | 6.3 |
| **Dried figs** | 5.6 | Cooked soybean | 1.6 |
| Guavas | 5.6 | Winter squash | 1.8 |
| Kale | 1.1 | Strawberries | 1.3 |
| Lentils | 1.6 | Walnuts | 1.7 |
| Okra | 1.0 | | |

**Date and Fig Juice Preparation**

Use pitted dates for easier juicing purposes. Wash under tap water (do not pat them dry with a towel; the extra water will make them juice better.) Do the same with figs, but cut off their stems before juicing. Dates and figs are incredibly sweet. Some wisdom and good judgment must be used as to the amount . It is better to double your date/fig concentrate with a little carrot juice. No more than half a cup of straight date/fig concentrate should be consumed at one time.

*Nice Fruit Laxative*

4 cups of boiling water
10½ Tbsp each of figs, raisins and uncooked barley
2¼ Tbsp cut dried licorice root

Directions: Simmer on low heat for 15 minutes then add licorice root. Remove from heat, permitting to steep for 30 minutes or so. When cold, stir and strain. Take one cup at night and again in the morning. Use a few raw figs to help any digestive disorder caused by eating too much red meat, fish, eggs, cheese or milk.

> **Please note that those who have blood sugar problems should not attempt to use these juices to relieve constipation.**

### Throat And Lung Problem Relief
Sore throat is an infection which is caused most commonly by viruses, bacteria, and fungi. Chronic drainage from allergies can also make your throat sore. Sometimes sore throats occur when stomach acid backs up into the esophagus and into the throat.

**Any sore throat that lasts more than a few days that is not relieved by gargling with warm salt water or figs, or has fever or a rash associated with it, demands the attention of your doctor.**

Once you determine the cause of your sore throat, nutrition can help. Bring two cups of water to a boil. Add 5¼ tablespoons of chopped figs. Simmer on low heat for five minutes. Cover and stir until cool. Sip half cupfuls every four hours or so to ease sore throat and lungs.

### Poultice For Sores And Boils
Put three to four figs in a pie tin with enough milk to cover them. Cover and place in an oven set on a very low temperature for one hour. By that time, the figs should have absorbed all the milk. Cut the figs open and lay them directly on the sore or boil. Using date/fig juice, which is very low in sugar content, can serve an equal purpose in promoting rapid healing of superficial wounds.

### Teeth Cleaning
Ripe figs cut in half are used to clean the teeth by rubbing the cut seeds against the enamel for several minutes.

### Arthritic Pain Relief
Arthritis means painful inflammation of a joint. The joint will be red, warm to the touch, and somewhat swollen. It can be caused by excessive calcium deposit, causing spurs or deposits of crystallized urine acids in the joints that irritate and cause pain. Arthritis is aggravated by an accumulation of toxic waste in the body. Arthritic tendencies can also be inherited.

*Rheumatoid Arthritis* is a chronic inflammatory disorder causing stiffness, deformity and pain of joints and muscles, redness, swelling, and decreased movement. It is an autoimmune disease where the body attacks itself and is self threatening. It can affect the lungs, blood vessels, spleen, and skin. Early signs include fatigue, muscular aches and pains, stiffness in the joints, and swelling.

*Osteoarthritis* is a wearing away ailment. Cartilage in joints waste away and calcium spurs may form on surfaces that have contact with bones.

*Bursitis* occurs around your larger joints where nature has provided a sack called a bursa. In the event of injury or overuse the sack can swell with fluid to act as an internal cushion or splint.

Sometimes these protective cushions become inflamed from the injury or excessive use. The area around the joint may be warm to the touch and even swollen and red.

*Gout*, which cases painful, red, swollen joints occurs more commonly in men of forty, but can affect women and younger people as well. Gout occurs when the body cannot get rid of uric acid, a waste product of protein. Your body rids itself of this uric acid through your kidneys, but sometimes the kidneys fail to do the job. Uric acid stays in your blood and in the fluid of your joints where it can cause trouble. When your joints become too rich in uric acid, crystals begin to form and inflame the joint, which becomes red, swollen, and quite painful.

Figs have a sulphur component which is valuable in the treatment of chronic joint inflammation and swelling of soft tissues common to rheumatoid arthritis and traumatic injuries, such as a twisted ankle or pulled muscle or ligament.

Soak about six figs in 1½ cups of water for a few minutes to soften them up slightly. Mash into a paste. Apply directly to any area of stiffness and soreness on the body. Cover with a heavy towel of warm flannel cloth and leave on for half an hour. It will bring incredible relief even on lower backaches.

## Protection Against Cancer

There are many different types of cancer. Some spread quickly and others take years to develop. The blood stream and the lymphatic system can take cancer cells to different parts of the body. Cancer is a severe disorder of the immune system where the replication process of the cells malfunctions, and cells reproduce wildly and invade the other organs and tissues. The basic causes of cancer are believed to be environmental, dietary and stress factors that allow normal cells to get out of control. Air pollution, pesticides, food additives, and drugs all contribute to the degree of health.

When you make figs part of your diet, you will store polyphenols in your body that act as antioxidants. Antioxidants destroy free radicals that damage your body and cause cancer. Adding 10 grams of fiber, or six figs, to your diet will slash the risk of *colon cancer*. Other anti-cancer agents found in figs include coumarins and benzaldehyde.

Jonathan L. Hartwell, a scientist with the National Cancer Institute, listed figs as a useful treatment for different kinds of cancer in his five-year survey. "Plants Used Against Cancer" published in the scientific journal *Llyodia* from 1967 to 1971. Hartwell's work has been compiled in a volume published by Quartermain Publishing. In 1978 a team of Japanese scientists led by Kochi identified benzaldehyde in a distillation of figs. The results were reported in Cancer Therapy Reports, National Institutes of Health, Volume 64, No. 1, pp. 21-23, 1980.

Figs can be a useful tool in the treatment of cancer when used with regular medical care and alternative therapies.

## Cholesterol Reduction

Cholesterol is a fat your body needs to help form certain hormones, cell membranes, and bile. Too much of this soft, waxy substance means trouble—it cannot dissolve in your blood. Cholesterol carries two types of lipoproteins: low-density lipoproteins (LDL) and high-density lipoproteins (HDL). LDL is "bad" cholesterol because it can build up on the walls of your arteries and form a hard deposit called plaque. Plaque can narrow your arteries so that your heart will have trouble pumping blood through them. A blood clot can also form near the plaque site. If it blocks the flow of blood to your heart, it can cause a heart attack. When a clot blocks the flow of blood to your brain, it can cause a stroke.

HDL cholesterol whisks cholesterol away from your arteries to your liver and eventually out of your body. This "good" cholesterol actually protects you from heart disease and stroke.

High cholesterol has no symptoms. You will never know that you have high cholesterol unless you get a blood test and learn your numbers. Total cholesterol over 240, LDL cholesterol over 160, and HDL cholesterol below 35 are dangerous levels. They could indicate an increased risk of heart disease. To lower your risk of high cholesterol, your total cholesterol should be below 200, LDL below 130, and HDL should be between 35 and 90.

If you eat more fiber, you will have a better cholesterol level. Figs contain fiber as well as polyphenols, plant compounds that act as an antioxidant. Polyphenols stop LDL cholesterol from building up in your arteries and they keep your blood cells from becoming sticky and clumping together.

### Stroke Threat Reduction

A stroke causes a loss of functioning brain tissue. There are two kinds of strokes: cerebral hemorrhage and cerebral thrombosis. Cerebral hemorrhage, caused by a weak blood vessel in the brain, is most probable with those having high blood pressure. It can also occur when arteries are clogged or weak.

Cerebral thrombosis is due to a clot or other blockage in a blood vessel in the brain. A mild attack can cause temporary confusion and light-headedness, difficulty in speaking clearly, weakness on one side of the body, vision dimness, confusion, severe speech difficulties, and/or sudden gradual loss or blurring of consciousness. A coma may result for short or long periods. Some early warnings of stroke which may only last for a few moments include one or more of the following symptoms:

- Fainting
- Stumbling
- Numbness
- Paralysis
- Blurring
- Seeing bright lights
- Loss of speech/memory

The triple punch of fiber, potassium and magnesium in figs means extra protection from strokes, especially if you have high blood pressure. More nutrient-rich fruits and vegetables should be your first line of defense.

### High Blood Pressure Reduction

High blood pressure is a disease involving the heart and arteries that carry fresh blood to every part of the body. It occurs when cholesterol deposits in walls of arteries harden and constrict blood vessels, compressing blood into a small volume and raising pressure. Emotional stress triggers blood pressure upward.

Hypertension is a major killer that causes strokes, heart disease, kidney disease, and more. It is a degenerative disease that can be reversed by changing your diet, exercising, and watching your weight. Figs provide potassium and calcium that are beneficial to people with high blood pressure. Both minerals, in combination with less sodium, keep your blood pressure under control. People who eat plenty of potassium-rich foods not only tend to have lower blood pressure, but also have less risk of related conditions like strokes. Potassium helps reduce high blood pressure in a number of ways: it helps prevent dangerous low density lipoprotein cholesterol from building up on artery walls; it helps to remove excess sodium from inside cells, keeping the body's fluid levels in balance and blood pressure in check. Fresh figs contain 348 mg of potassium, 10 percent of the daily value (DV), and dried figs are even better with these figs providing 399 mg, 11 percent of DV.

## Diabetes Control

Diabetes mellitus is a metabolic disorder with abnormally high blood glucose levels. Symptoms include excessive thirst and urination, frequent and excessive hunger, weakness, depression, skin disorder, bowel and vaginal infections, blurred vision, tingling leg cramps, impotence, dry mouth, numbness in feet/hands.

Juvenile diabetes (Type I) called Insulin Dependent Diabetes Mellitus (IDDM) causes the pancreas to produce no insulin, the hormone responsible for moving the sugar in the blood into the cell. This is the more serious type of diabetes, and almost always develops in childhood.

Adult diabetes (Type II) causes the pancreas to produce insulin, but the cells have too few chemical receptions and the cells starve, resulting in lack of energy. The major cause of Type II diabetes is thought to be obesity. Overeating and eating the wrong kinds of foods are the major cause of diabetes.

If you are worried about high blood sugar, look no further than the fig. Figs are not a high-carb food. Fiber in figs will lower your glucose. Fiber slows the amount of glucose your body absorbs from your small intestine. High fiber diet, 50 grams per day, helps keep blood sugar, insulin, and cholesterol under control. Eating and chewing delicious figs is a tasty way to get more fiber.

## Weight Loss

Fiber can help you lose weight, which will not only shrink your waistline, but also your risk of heart disease and other health problems too. Figs are filling; therefore, you would eat less if you ate more figs—they stay in your stomach longer. They are not super-high in calories or fat either. You will get just 48 calories and almost no fat in every dried fruit.

## Kidney, Bladder Infection Reduction

If you have kidney stones, oxalate is an enemy. Oxalate is found in foods such as spinach, tomatoes, cranberries, rhubarb, peanuts, coffee, tea and chocolate. However, calcium keeps your body from absorbing oxalate, and you are less likely to form oxalate-based kidney stones. Do not load up on calcium supplements as you might actually increase your risk of calcium-based kidney stones. Get calcium through whole foods. Eating 10 dried figs gives you 33 percent of the recommended dietary allowance of calcium. You may stave off kidney stones as well with the potassium in dried figs. More potassium means less risk of kidney stones. Ten dried figs provide more than half your daily potassium needs.

## Corns And Warts Control

Figs contain protein-dissolving enzymes that might help soften and eliminate corns (a corny and thickened area of the skin which may be either soft or hard depending on its location on the foot due to pressure or friction). Fig latex contains ficin, which is a strong remedy for treating corns. Break a fig leaf from its branch and let the latex (white sap) drop onto the affected area.

**Celiac Diseases**
Figs can eliminate celiac disease, also called sprue.
Celiac sprue is a chronic intestinal disorder in
which intolerance to gluten, a protein found in
grains (especially wheat), interferes with the proper
absorption of many nutrients. Figs contain unique
protein carbohydrates, complex and mineral salts,
which halt an abnormal response started by gluten
in the small intestine.

**Insomnia Relief**
The consumption of carbohydrate rich foods
towards bedtime will quite often induce sleep.
A little date/fig juice may be the perfect
nightcap for an insomniac, unless there are
blood-sugar problems.

# Chapter Three

# THE NUTRIENT RICH FIG

Why is the fig a miracle fruit? Humans have eaten figs since the millennia, and figs have been a staple in the diets of many ancient cultures. Today we know that the fig is a healing fruit because of its many nutrients.

**Potassium**

Although the vast majority of potassium remains inside your body cells, a small amount remains outside. That small amount is of critical importance in contributing to the passage of electrical nerve impulses throughout the body and controlling the contraction of muscles, including heart muscles. Potassium also helps to maintain your blood pressure.

Certain diuretic medication causes your kidneys to rid your body of excess fluid by making you waste sodium, such as thiazides (hydrochlorothiozide) and farosemide (lasix,

bumex) causing a pumping, not only of sodium, but also of potassium. Caffeine, as well as certain diuretics and heart/blood pressure medications, causes you to waste more potassium through your kidneys. *Symptoms of Deficiency:*

- Acne
- Constipation
- Salt and fluid retention
- Stunted growth
- Low blood pressure
- Fatigue
- Insomnia
- Muscle weakness and cramping
- Thirst
- Depression
- Nervousness
- Clouded thinking
- Sugar intolerance
- High cholesterol

- Extremely dry skin and mouth
- Heart palpitations

Figs are especially rich in potassium, although other foods, including dried apricots, cantaloupes, lima beans, potatoes, avocados, bananas, broccoli, milk, peanut butter, and citrus fruits are good sources as well.

## Calcium

Calcium is the fifth most abundant mineral in the human body. The miracle fruit, the fig, is rich in calcium. Other food sources include dairy products, broccoli, kale, spinach, collard and turnip greens, cabbage, cauliflower, asparagus, egg yolks, beans, lentils, nuts, and tofu.

The major role of calcium is in maintaining integrity of the skeletal system. Calcium also plays a critical role in the coagulation of blood, in the generation and transmission of nerve impulses; in the contraction of muscle fibers; in the activation of certain enzyme systems; and in the relationship of some hormones. Vitamin D is required for adequate absorption of calcium from the gastrointestinal tract. Stress and immobilization can reduce your ability to absorb calcium from the gastrointestinal tract. Cocoa, soybeans, and carbonated cola also interfere with the absorption of calcium, as well as protein in the diet. Caffeine increases the loss of calcium through the kidneys. Iron may enhance the absorption of calcium.

*Symptoms of Deficiency:*

- Agitation
- Hyperactivity
- Nervousness and irritability
- Brittle fingernails
- Insomnia
- High blood pressure
- Localized numbness and tingling sensations
- Numbness of an appendage

- Muscle cramps or even tetany (grabbing or locking spasms)
- Clouded or confused thinking
- Delusions
- Depression
- Heart palpitations
- Stunted growth
- Disease of the gums and tooth support structure
- Tooth decay

## Phosphorus

Phosphorus is a mineral that occurs widely in nature, especially in figs. Other food sources include milk, eggs, grains, nuts, dried beans, peas, lentils, and green leafy vegetables.

Phosphorus, along with calcium, gives strength to your bones and teeth. It assists in a variety of chemical reactions in the body; energy production; metabolism of protein, carbohydrates and fat; and contributes protein. Antacids, which contains either magnesium or aluminum, can interfere with your ability to absorb phosphorus. Iron can also interfere with your ability to absorb phosphorous. Calcium and phosphorous exist in a balance in your bones and teeth. If you eat a diet containing too much phosphorus, your body's tendency to balance these two minerals could cause calcium to be pulled from the bones, weakening them. Normal phosphorus metabolism requires sufficient amounts of vitamin D.

*Symptoms of Deficiency:*

- Loss of appetite
- Weight loss
- Weakness and fatigue
- Numbness and tingling sensations
- Bone pain
- Anxiety
- Apprehension

## Magnesium

Nearly seventy percent of the body's supply of magnesium is found in the bones, with about thirty percent in body fluids and in the muscle and soft tissue. Figs are a major contributor to body magnesium. Other food sources include whole seeds such as nuts and legumes, wheat germ, green vegetables, spinach, soybeans, peas, molasses, and cornmeal.

Magnesium functions in a critical capacity as a contractor or coenzyme in energy production and the metabolism of glucose and the oxidation of fatty acids. It is involved in protein synthesis and the transmission of the genetic message through productions of DNA and RNA. A high-fat diet can reduce magnesium absorption because the fat and magnesium combine to form soap-like compounds that the gastrointestinal tract cannot absorb. A high fiber diet can promote loss of some minerals. A deficiency of Vitamin E may reduce magnesium levels in the tissues. Alcohol, potassium, and caffeine all decrease magnesium through the kidneys. High sugar intake increases your need for magnesium. Balance your calcium intake with magnesium. You need more magnesium if your blood cholesterol levels are high.

*Symptoms of Deficiency:*
- Anemia
- Loss of appetite
- Heart rhythm disturbances
- Agitation
- Anxiety
- Confusion
- Depression
- Disorientation
- Hallucinations
- Hyperactivity
- Irritability
- Nervousness
- Restlessness
- Jumpiness
- Neurological symptoms including numbness and tingling
- Difficulty balancing while walking
- Muscular symptoms including, tremors, pains and weakness

## Iron

Your body needs iron to produce hemoglobin, the oxygen-carrying pigment that makes red blood cells red. It is a helper for a variety of important enzymes that are necessary for good health. Other food sources include eggs, spinach, asparagus, prunes, raisins, cream of wheat, and dried apricots. You need iron to make healthy blood cells. Iron helps to produce your immune defense white blood cells. Excess calcium competes with iron in your intestine. Excess iron reduces your ability to absorb copper and zinc. Coffee and tea may reduce your ability to absorb iron. Medications like Tagamet, Zantac, Pepcid, and Axid may reduce your ability to absorb iron. Milk may also reduce your ability to absorb iron. You must have adequate amounts of the B vitamins to absorb and use iron properly. Deficiency of Vitamin A reduces your ability to absorb iron.

*Symptoms of Deficiency:*
- Anemia
- Cracking mouth
- Inflamed tongue
- Loss of appetite
- Fragile bones
- Sensitivity to the cold
- Constipation
- Confusion
- Dizziness
- Difficulty swallowing

- Fatigue
- Brittle nails
- Headaches

## Copper

Copper is component of several enzymes stimulating iron absorption. Other food sources include nuts, seeds, cherries, and coca. Copper works in concert with iron. It is needed to make blood cells, connective tissues, and nerve fibers. Copper is the chief structural protein of your body and promotes production in skin pigment. Alcohol may worsen the deficiency of copper. Egg yolks can bind with copper in your intestine and prevent its absorption. Iron may reduce your ability to absorb copper from your intestinal tract. Vitamin C in high doses can decrease your absorption of copper from food.

*Symptoms of Deficiency:*

- Spotty hair loss
- Anemia
- Rashes
- Emphysema
- Fatigue
- High cholesterol
- Frequent infections
- Depression
- Heart muscle damage
- Osteoporosis

## Manganese

Manganese is needed for normal tendon and bone structure. Figs are a major source of system manganese. Other food sources include whole grains and cereal, fruits, green vegetables, dried legumes, ginger, clover, and nuts.

Your body needs manganese to metabolize fat properly; to build bones and connective tissues;

and to produce energy. If you overload on iron you will impair your ability to absorb manganese.

*Symptoms of Deficiency:*

- Fragile bones
- Rashes
- Sugar intolerance
- High cholesterol
- Nausea
- Weight loss

## Fiber

Fibers are the parts of plant foods that are not absorbed in the human digestive tract. Fiber's value in normal digestive function has been recognized for centuries. It is an important component of the human diet. We should process no fewer than 15 grams and no more than 35 grams of fiber a day. It should come from moderate amounts of a variety of fruits, vegetables, and grains and not from pills. *What is Dietary Fiber?* Almost all fibers are complex carbohydrates, except lignin. The human digestive tract lacks the enzymes to break down these carbohydrates into a form that can be absorbed and used for energy.

Fibers are classified as either soluble or insoluble. The soluble fibers are those that are sticky and mesh with water to form gels. Insoluble fibers are those that pass through the digestive tract much unchanged except for being altered by chewing. They absorb large amounts of water (up to 15 times their weight), thus creating a soft bulky stool. The typical diet of most industrialized countries is high in animal products, sugar, and processed foods that have little or no fiber. There are many different varieties of fiber, and all are good in moderation. Eat a wide variety of fruits, vegetables and grains (as you can afford), adding up to a total of 24 to 35 grams of fiber per day.

## Soluble Dietary Fibers

| Type of Fiber | Sources | Functions |
|---|---|---|
| Cellulose | Bran, whole grains, nuts, white part of orange rind | Add bulk to stool to reduce constipation, diverticulosis, hemorrhoids |
| Pectin | Legumes, apples, figs, pears, other fruits and nuts | Lower blood cholesterol, normalize blood sugar |
| Mucilage | Plant seeds, plant secretions | Lower blood cholesterol, normalize blood sugar |
| Guar, carrageen | Algae and seaweed | Lower blood cholesterol, normalize blood sugar |
| Lignin | Woody part of bran, fruit skin, whole grains | Lower blood cholesterol, normalize blood sugar |
| Hemi cellulose | Vegetables, fruits, nuts, whole grains | Add bulk to stool to reduce constipation, diverticulosis, hemorrhoids |

## Effects of Fiber

*Bowel Function:* Fiber, especially cellulose and hemicelluloses, act as tiny spoons, absorbing many times their weight in water. As a result, feces become soft, and bulky. This bulky stool stimulates peristalsis, the rhythmic contraction of the bowel, thus passes more easily and rapidly through the digestive tract. This helps prevent constipation and related problems due to increased intestinal pressure, such as diverticulosis and hemorrhoids.

*Diverticulosis Disease:* Caused by the formation of small out pouches of packets in weakened segment of the intestinal wall. Excessive pressure within the colon worsens the condition by further weakening the pockets and forcing waste material into them. There is a danger that the pockets will rupture, thus spilling bowel contents into the pelvic cavity, causing serious infection. A high fiber regimen can halt this progression and erase symptoms.

*Irritable Bowel Syndrome:* Spasmodic contractions of the bowel muscles, resulting in abdominal pain, gas, and alternating diarrhea and constipation. A high fiber diet is frequently recommended.

*Colon Cancer:* Colon cancer may be caused by prolonged contact with carcinogens in the stool since the stool produced by a low fiber diet travels more and more slowly through the colon than one high in fiber. Figs have a definite laxative effect on the body and may be helpful in avoiding colon disease.

*Heart Disease:* Certain types of fiber may reduce the chances of heart attacks, specifically the developing of coronary arteriosclerosis. There is sound evidence that soluble fiber can have cholesterol lowering effects.

Food Value per 100 grams of Edible Protein

| Nutrient Element | Fresh Figs | Dried |
|---|---|---|
| Calories | 80 | 274 |
| Moisture | 77.5 – 86.8g | 23g |
| Protein | 1.2 – 1.3g | 4.3g |
| Fat | 0.14 – 0.30g | 1.3g |
| Carbohydrates | 17.1 – 20.3g | 69.1g |
| Fiber | 1.2 – 2.2g | 5.6g |
| Ash | 0.48 – 0.85g | 2.3g |
| Calcium | 35 – 78.2mg | 126mg |
| Phosphorus | 22 – 32.9mg | 77mg |
| Iron | 0.6 – 4.09mg | 3.0mg |
| Sodium | 2.0mg | 34mg |
| Potassium | 194mg | 640.mg |
| Carotene | 0.013 – 0.195mg | -- |
| Vitamin A | 20 – 270 I.V. | 80. I.V. |
| Thiamin | 0.034 – 0.06mg | 0.10mg |
| Riboflavin | 0.053 – 0.079mg | 0.10mg |
| Niacin | 0.32 – 0.412mg | 0.7mg |
| Ascorbic Acid | 12.2 – 17.6mg | -- |
| Citric Acid | 0.10 – 0.44mg | -- |

## General Nutrient Values of Figs

| Fig | Serving Size | Calories | Grams | | | | |
|---|---|---|---|---|---|---|---|
| | | | Protein | Carbs | Sodium | Fiber | Fat |
| Candied | 100 g | 299 | 3.5 | 73.7 | 34 | >5.6c | 0.2 |
| **Raw** | 1 large | 47 | 0.5 | 12.3 | 1 | 2.1 | 0.2 |
| Trimmed | 1 oz. | 21 | 0.2 | 5.4 | 61 | >.3c | |
| Canned in extra heavy syrup | 4 oz. | 121 | 0.4 | 31.6 | 1 | >.6c | 0.1 |
| In heavy syrup | 4 oz. | 100 | 0.4 | 26.0 | 1 | >.6c | 0.1 |
| In light syrup | 4 oz. | 78 | 0.4 | 20.0 | 1 | >.6c | 0.1 |
| In water | 4 oz. | 60 | 0.5 | 15.9 | 1 | >.6c | 0.1 |
| **Dried** | 1 large | 47.7 | 0.57 | 12.2 | 2.1 | 1.8 | 0.2 |
| Cooked | 4 oz. | 122 | 1.5 | 31.3 | 6 | >2.3c | 0.6 |
| Stewed | ½ cup | 140 | 1.7 | 35.8 | 7 | 6.2 | 0.6 |
| Uncooked | 4 oz. | 289 | 3.5 | 74.1 | 15 | 10.5 | 1.3 |
| Uncooked | 1 cup | 507 | 6.1 | 130.1 | 22 | 18.5 | 2.3 |
| Uncooked Calimyrna | ½ cup | 250 | 3.0 | 58.0 | 10 | (mg) | 2.0 |
| Uncooked Mission | ½ cup | 210 | 3.0 | 1.0 | 20 | (mg) | (mg) |
| Uncooked Trimmed | 10 fruits | 477 | 5.7 | 122.2 | 21 | 17.4 | 2.2 |

## Vitamin and Mineral Values in Figs

| Fig Type | No. | A IU | Thi Mg | Rib Mg | Nia mg | B6 mg | Fol mcg | B12 mcg | C mg | Cal mg | Iron mg | Mag mg | Pot mg | Zn Mg |
|---|---|---|---|---|---|---|---|---|---|---|---|---|---|---|
| Candied | 100gm | 80 | 0.1 | 0.1 | .7 | N/A | N/A | N/A | 0.0 | 126.0 | 3.0 | N/A | 640.6 | N/A |
| Raw | 1 large | 91 | .04 | .03 | 0.26 | .07 | N/A | 0 | 1.3 | 22.4 | 0.24 | 10.48 | 148.88 | 0.1 |
| Canned in extra heavy syrup | 1 cup | 94 | .06 | .09 | 1.09 | N/A | N/A | 0 | 2.6 | 67.86 | .73 | 26.1 | 253.17 | 0.26 |
| In heavy syrup | 1 cup | 96 | .06 | 0.1 | 1.11 | N/A | N/A | 0 | 2.6 | 69.93 | .73 | 25.9 | 256.41 | .28 |
| In light syrup | 1 cup | 93 | .06 | 0.1 | 1.1 | N/A | N/A | 0 | 2.5 | 68.04 | .73 | 25.2 | 257.04 | .28 |
| In water | 1 cup | 94 | .06 | .08 | 1.1 | N/A | N/A | 0 | 2.5 | 96.44 | .73 | 24.4 | 255.44 | .03 |
| Dried | 1 large | 25 | 0.013 | 0.016 | 0.13 | 0.042 | 1.4 | 0 | 0.015 | 26.9 | 0.41 | 11.1 | 133.1 | 0.095 |
| Stewed | ½ cup | 207 | 0.1 | .14 | .83 | .17 | 1.3 | 0 | 5.7 | 79.3 | 1.22 | 35.5 | 391.3 | .27 |
| Uncooked | 1 cup | 265 | .13 | .18 | 1.38 | .45 | 14.9 | 0 | 1.6 | 286.56 | 4.44 | 117.41 | 1416.83 | 1.01 |
| Uncooked Trimmed | 10 fruits | 249 | .13 | .16 | 1.3 | .42 | 14.0 | 0 | 1.5 | 269.28 | 4.17 | 110.33 | 1331.44 | .95 |

### Read More About Figs in Diet and Health

Carlson, Wade. <u>Inner Cleansing: How to Free Yourself from Joint-Muscle-Artery-Circulation Sludge.</u> Prentice Hall Trade, 1992.

Hartnell, Jonathan L. <u>Plants Used Against Cancer</u>. Quartermain Publications, 1982.

Heinerman, John. <u>Heinerman's Encyclopedia of Healing Juices</u>. Prentice Hall Press, 1994.

Margen, Sheldon. <u>The Wellness Encyclopedia of Food & Nutrition.</u> Random House, 1992.

Tenney, Louise. <u>Nutritional Guide With Food Combining.</u> Woodland Publishing. 1994.

## Chapter Four

# CLASSIC FIG RECIPES

**Shopping for Figs**

Figs, whether fresh or dried, should be firm, but still yield slightly to the touch. If dried figs are rock hard, do not buy them. If fresh figs seem mushy, they are too ripe and will not deliver full flavor. Healthy figs and ripe mission figs will always have a rich color. Look for shapely, plump figs with unbruised, unbroken skins and a mild fragrance (sour smelling figs indicate spoilage). Figs should be just soft to the touch, but not mushy. When buying packages of dried figs, check for unbroken wrapping. The figs should give slightly when gently squeezed through the package. String figs, imported from Greece from October through December, should be firm and clean. Obvious things to avoid are blemishes, shrivel, rot, mushiness, fermented odor, and puddles of juice. Fresh figs deteriorate rapidly, usually within a few days. They will stay fresh for about three days when stored in the refrigerator. Dried figs, by contrast, will keep for months when stored in an airtight bag in the refrigerator.

**Preparation**

Figs, both fresh and dried, are easy to handle. Some people peel the skin from the stem end to expose the flesh for eating by hand. The more fastidious eater holds the fruit by the stem end, cuts the fruit into quarters from the apex, spreads the section apart, lifts the flesh from the skin with a knife blade and discards the stem and skin. Commercially, figs are peeled by immersion for one minute in boiling lye water or a boiling solution of sodium bicarbonate. In warm, humid, climates figs are eaten without peeling and served with cream and sugar.

Peeled or unpeeled, figs may be merely stewed or cooked in various ways (pies, pudding, cakes, bread, other bakery products), added to ice cream mixes, jam, marmalade, paste and compotes. Fig paste forms the filling of well-known Fig Newton's. They are sometimes commercially can-dried.

Because figs are extremely sticky, they can be difficult to eat. Chilling the figs for an hour before cutting will help prevent them from sticking to the knife or scissors. The flavor and fragrance of fresh figs are best, however, at room temperature. Simply quarter the figs lengthwise and place them on a plate. A sprinkle of orange or lemon juice will heighten their flavor.

Figs also work well with walnuts or almonds. Use dried figs in recipes that can replace apricots, dates, or other fruit. Try them in whole-wheat muffins, cookies and cake fillings. Stir chopped dried figs into low-fat cream cheese and spread on pumpernickel bread, or mix figs into cottage cheese and serve with crackers. Sweeten cooked cereal by adding chopped figs during the last minute of cooking time. Chopping dried figs provides an interesting texture to fresh fruit salads; combine them with bananas or berries. For a special vegetable side dish, sprinkle chopped dried figs over baked sweet potatoes or winter squash, or stir the figs into mashed sweet potatoes or in squash. Thread skewers with fresh or dried figs and grill with kebabs, or offer them on their own as a barbecue dessert.

## APPETIZERS, SAUCES, AND SALADS

### Colonel's Fig Chutney and Fig Puree

1½ cups (8 ounces) California figs, stems removed
1 tablespoon grated fresh ginger
1 cup fruit-flavored vinegar (raspberry, blueberry, or mango) or white wine or cider vinegar
1 whole lime, coarsely chopped

¼ teaspoon red pepper flakes or dash hot pepper sauce
1 medium onion, chopped
3 to 4 cloves garlic, minced

Halve or quarter figs, or leave whole. In a medium saucepan, combine figs with all remaining ingredients. Cover and simmer until figs are very soft, about 30 minutes. Uncover and simmer until thick and syrupy, about 15 minutes. Serve with meat, fish or poultry, or stir into mayonnaise to make a salad dressing or sauce. Makes about 2 cups.

### Fig Purée

1½ cups (8 ounces) California figs
1 teaspoon vanilla
1/3 cup fruit juice (orange, lemon, lime, pineapple, cranberry or any blend) or water
½ to 1 teaspoon cinnamon
½ teaspoon nutmeg

Combine in blender or food processor and mix until puréed. Cover and refrigerate. Makes about 2 cups.

### Stuffed Fig Appetizers

**Brie Stuffed Figs with Fresh Rosemary**
Remove stems and slice open one side of each fig. Stuff with a small piece of Brie or Camembert cheese and chopped fresh rosemary leaves. Sprinkle with freshly ground black pepper. Place cheese-side up in baking pan. Bake at 350° F for 7 minutes or until hot.

**Chutney-Ham Stuffed Figs**
Remove stems and cut open figs. Stuff with

a small cube of deli-smoked ham and a dab of chopped chutney. Garnish with herb sprig.

**Bacon-Wrapped Fruited Figs**
Bake bacon at 400° F for 10 minutes or until bacon is cooked but still flexible. Cut strips in half. Remove stems and cut open figs. Stuff with a small chunk of fresh peach, nectarine or mango. Wrap with half-slice bacon (may not

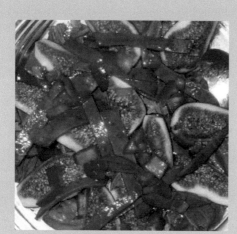
*Fresh Figs with Prosciutto*

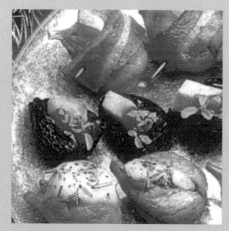
*Stuffed Fig Appetizers*

entirely go around fig) and fasten with pick. Bake at 400° F for 7 minutes or until hot.

**Sherry Cheese Stuffed Figs**
Remove stems and cut open figs. Beat ½ cup garlic-herb cheese spread with 2 teaspoons sherry or white wine. Spoon into figs. Garnish with fresh thyme leaves.

**Hawaiian-Style Stuffed Figs**
Remove stems and cut open figs. Stuff with a small cube of fresh or canned pineapple. Wrap fig with thinly-sliced prosciutto, making a band around center of fig. Sprinkle with toasted sesame seeds.

*Fig Fruit Basket Salad Dressing*

½ cup finely chopped California dried figs
1 cup orange or peach yogurt
1 (8¼ ounce) can crushed pineapple, drained
1/8 teaspoon nutmeg

Combine figs with yogurt, pineapple and nutmeg; chill until serving time. Spoon over fruit salad. Makes 6 to 8 servings.

*Fennel, Orange and Fig Salad*

2 small fennel bulbs, thinly sliced
2 seedless oranges, peeled and separated into sections
4 fresh figs, quartered or 8 dried mission figs, soaked in hot water to cover until soft, about 30 minutes, drained then quartered
¼ cup chopped oil-cured black olives
2 Tbsp extra virgin olive oil
1 juice of lime
3 tsp whole fennel seeds

Salt and freshly ground black pepper to taste

Directions: Cut the sliced fennel into 1 inch pieces. Arrange an equal number of fennel and orange slices on each serving plate. Arrange the figs on top. Sprinkle with an even amount of olives. In a blender or food processor, or using an immersion blender, beat together the olive oil and lime juice to make a thick emulsion. Add the fennel seeds and salt and pepper. Stir well. Pour a spoonful over each serving.

### Warm Figs Goat Cheese

24 small fresh black figs, halved lengthwise
¾ cup crumbled goat cheese or try other grated melting cheese such as aged provolone or ranchero
1½ Tbsp balsamic vinegar
Freshly ground black pepper

Directions: Preheat oven to 350° F. Arrange the figs on a baking sheet, cut sides up. Spoon a little goat cheese on each fig half. Lightly brush the figs with the vinegar and sprinkle the cheese with pepper. Bake for about 8 minutes or until the figs are warmed through. Transfer the figs to a platter and serve immediately

### Fruited Dressing

*California figs add the sweetness and flavor to this easy fruit topper. Try the dressing over whatever fruit is in season—citrus in winter, berries in the spring, peaches and plums in summer, apples and pears in the fall. It's also great over sliced chicken, roast beef or pork.*

½ cup lemon or limejuice
2 Tbsp walnut oil
6 California figs, stems removed

Dash salt
3 tablespoons fruit-flavored vinegar

Combine all ingredients in blender or food processor and blend until smooth. Serve over mixed fruit, toss with assorted greens or drizzle over grilled chicken or tuna atop assorted greens. Makes about 2/3 cup.

### Fig Tapenade

½ lb ripe black figs
2 Tbsp drained capers
2 Tbsp sugar
1 tsp dried tarragon
6 canned anchovy fillet, drained
2 Tbsp extra virgin olive oil
¾ cup drained pitted calamata olives, coarsely chopped

Directions: Rinse figs, trim off and discard stems. Coarsely chop figs. In a 1 to 2 quart pan over medium-high heat, combine figs, sugar and one tablespoon water. Stir occasionally until mixture is boiling gently and figs turn shiny and darker (3 to 5 minutes). In a food processor or a blender, whirl fig mixture, olives, anchovies, capers, tarragon and olive oil until coarsely pureed, scraping mixture into a small bowl.

### Fresh Figs with Prosciutto

1½ oz argali
1 Tbsp fresh orange juice
4 fresh figs
1 Tbsp clear honey
4 slice proscuitto
1 small red chili
4 Tbsp olive oil

Directions: Tear argali into fairly small pieces and arrange on 4 serving plates. Using a sharp knife, cut each fig into quarters. Place them on top of the argali leaves. Using a sharp knife, cut the prosciutto into strips and scatter over the argali and figs. Place the oil, orange juice, and honey in a screw-top jar. Shake the jar vigorously until the mixture emulsifies and forms a thick dressing. Transfer to a serving bowl. Using a sharp knife, dice the chili. Add the chopped chili to the dressing and mix well. Drizzle the dressing over the prosciutto, argali, and figs. Toss to mix well. *Chilies can burn the skin for several hours after chopping, so it is advisable to wear gloves when you are handling the hot varieties.

### Fig Chutney

Can be served hot, sour or spicy, smooth or chunky. All use sugar and vinegar as preservatives.
5 cups red wine vinegar
½ lb pitted dates coarsely chopped
1 lb light brown sugar
¼ cup finely shredded fresh ginger
2 tsp salt
2 tsp sweet paprika
1 lb onions, sliced into three rings
1 tsp white mustard seed
2 lb firm, slightly under ripe, black figs (sliced into ½" thick rounds)
3 tsp chopped fresh tarragon or
1 tsp. dried tarragon

Directions: Put the vinegar, sugar and salt in a non-corrosive saucepan, stirring until the sugar is dissolved. Bring to a boil and then simmer for about 5 minutes. Add the fig, onions, dates, and spices; bring to a boil then simmer for one hour until the mixture is thick and most of the liquid evaporates. Remove the pan from the heat and stir in the tarragon. Ladle into the hot sterilized jars, then seal. The chutney will be ready to eat in one month.

### Fig Pickles

1 Tbsp baking soda
1 pint vinegar
1 gallon water
½ Tbsp cloves
1 lb fresh figs
3 lemons, sliced thin
3 lb sugar

Directions: Dissolve soda in water. Heat to boiling and pour over figs. Let stand a few minutes. Drain and rinse thoroughly in cold water. Dissolve sugar in vinegar. Add cinnamon cloves and lemons. Heat to boiling. Add figs and cool until clear. Leave out figs and pack in jars. Boil down vinegar syrup until thick and pour over figs.

### Fig Basket Salad Dressing

½ cup finely chopped California dried figs
1 cup orange or peach yogurt
1 (8¼ ounce) can crushed pineapple, drained
1/8 teaspoon nutmeg

Combine figs with yogurt, pineapple and nutmeg; chill until serving time. Spoon over fruit salad. Makes 6 to 8 servings

### Company Fig Cheese Spread

4 oz. low-fat sharp cheddar cheese
¼ cup chunked red bell pepper (or substitute 2 Tbsp canned pimento)
4 oz. non-fat ricotta cheese

½ cup walnuts
1 clove garlic
½ cup California Dried Figs
2 tablespoons low or non-fat milk
¼ cup parsley sprigs

If using a food processor, cut low-fat cheddar cheese into cubes. Process until finely chopped. Add ricotta cheese, process about 10 seconds. Add remaining ingredients, except milk, and process until all ingredients are finely chopped. Add milk as needed to reach desired consistency. Serve with crackers or crisp vegetable sticks. Makes about 2 cups.

## FIGS FOR DINNER

### Fresh Figs with Smithfield Ham and Mustard Cream

¼ cup crème fraise or sour cream
¼ cup heavy cream
2 tsp Creole mustard or whole-grain mustard
8 ripe figs (white figs) gently washed, dried, stems trimmed
¼ lb Julienne Smithfield ham
About 1 cup loosely packed freshly ground black pepper, to taste
Fresh mint sprigs to garnish

Directions: Place garnish in a small bowl. Combine crème fraise, cream and mustard. Divide sauce evenly among four medium salad plates. Cut each fig in half through the stem end. Gently stuff fig halves with all but 2 or 4 tablespoons of the ham. Place 4 fig halves out side up with stem ends pointing toward the center on the mustard cream on each plate. Sprinkle with remaining ham and pepper to taste. Garnish with mint, if desired.

### Spinach Salad with Stuffed Figs & Warm Port Dressing

1 cup packed Blue Ribbon Orchard Choice or Sun-Maid Mission or Calimyrna figs
2 teaspoons Dijon mustard
Salt and ground black pepper
½ cup port
2 tablespoons olive oil
1 teaspoon sugar
12 ounces baby spinach leaves, stems removed
1½ teaspoons finely chopped fresh rosemary
2 tablespoons goat cheese
½ cup (2 oz.) thin strips prosciutto
3 tablespoons finely chopped, roasted pistachios
¼ cup thinly sliced red onion
2 tablespoons balsamic vinegar

Remove fig stems. Starting at the stem end, cut an "X" three-quarters of way to bottom of 8 figs. Finely chop remaining figs. In small saucepan, combine whole and chopped figs, port, shallot, sugar and rosemary. Cover and bring to boil; reduce heat and simmer 1 minute. Remove from heat and set aside for 10 minutes. Moisten hands

*Spinach Salad with Stuffed Figs*

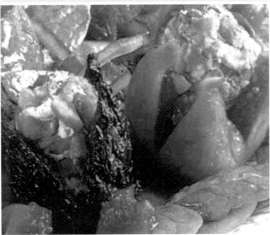

with water and form goat cheese into 8 small balls. Roll in nuts. Cover and chill until serving time. To fig-port mixture, add balsamic vinegar, mustard, salt and pepper to taste. Stir in olive oil. Heat dressing just until warm. Combine spinach, prosciutto and red onion in large bowl. Remove whole figs from dressing and reserve; toss remaining dressing and chopped figs with salad. Place salad on 4 small plates. Fill whole figs with cheese balls and arrange on plates. Makes 4 servings.

### *Rice Frittata with Figs and Parmesan Cheese*

½ cup finely chopped onion
¾ oz. parmesan cheese, freshly grated
½ small garlic clove, minced
¼ teaspoon dried thyme
2 eggs + 3 egg whites
2 teaspoons olive oil
½ cup cooked white rice
2 large dried California figs, finely chopped

Spray medium nonstick saucepan with nonstick cooking spray; place over medium heat 30 seconds. Add onion and garlic; sauté until soft, 5 minutes. In large bowl, beat eggs and egg whites; stir in the rice, the onion mixture, the figs, cheese and thyme. Return skillet to medium-high heat 30 seconds. Add oil; heat 30 seconds more. Pour in egg-rice mixture and cook until lightly browned on bottom, about 3-4 minutes. Slide onto large plate, then invert plate onto skillet to brown other side, 2-3 minutes.

### *Savory Fig Stuffing Balls*

¾ cup chopped onion
4 cups cubed herb-seasoned dry
bread stuffing mix
½ cup chopped celery

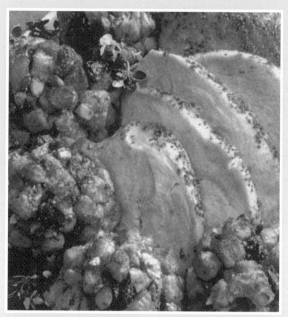
*Savory Fig Stuffing Balls*

¼ cup chopped carrot
½ cup chopped toasted almonds
3 tablespoons butter, divided
1/3 cup chopped fresh parsley
1 cup chopped Blue Ribbon Orchard Choice or Sun-Maid Mission or Calimyrna Figs
1/3 to 2/3 cup chicken broth
Salt and ground black pepper, to taste
½ cup chopped, cooked smoked lean sausage
1 large egg, lightly beaten
¾ cup dry sherry or chicken broth

Heat oven to 350° F. In large deep skillet or Dutch oven, stir and cook onion, celery, and carrot in 1 tablespoon butter over medium heat until onion is soft. Stir in figs, sausage and sherry; simmer for 2 minutes. Remove from heat and stir in bread cubes, nuts, parsley and 1/3 cup chicken broth. Add salt and pepper, to taste. Stir in egg. Form mounded ½ cup portions of stuffing into balls, packing tightly and moistening with additional chicken broth if needed. Place on greased baking sheet. Melt remaining butter and brush on balls. Bake 25 to 30 minutes, until hot and golden. Makes 8 to 10 balls.

### Fig Ranch Style Chops

6 lean pork steaks or chops
2 tablespoons brown sugar
Salt and pepper
½ teaspoon cinnamon
6 California dried figs, sliced
1 tablespoon apple mint jelly
1 tart apple, cored and sliced

Place meat in large shallow baking dish. Season with salt and pepper. Top with dried figs and apples. Sprinkle with brown sugar and cinnamon. Dot each chop with a dab of jelly. Bake, covered, for 40 minutes at 350° F. Uncover and bake an additional 20 minutes. Makes 6 servings.

### Fig & Rosemary Focaccia

*These Mediterranean flavors prove they were made for each other. Start with brown-and-serve focaccia, or pre-baked from scratch or frozen bread dough. This simple bread can turn a broiled chicken breast and salad into an elegant meal!*

1 cup California figs, stems removed
¼ cup fresh rosemary leaves
¼ cup fruity olive oil
1 10-inch focaccia
Zest and juice of 1 lemon
Kosher salt

Add figs, oil, lemon zest and juice and rosemary to food processor container and process until figs and rosemary are finely chopped. Place focaccia on baking sheet and spread fig mixture over top. Sprinkle lightly with salt. Bake in preheated 375° F oven until browned, about 10 to 15 minutes. Cut wedges to serve. Makes 6 to 8 servings

### Fig Maple Glazed Ham Steak

1 fully cooked ham steak (1 to 1½ inches thick)
1 tablespoon melted butter
Powdered cloves
8 California dried figs, halved
1/3 cup maple-flavored syrup
2 bananas, peeled and quartered
1 tablespoon lemon juice

Slash edges of ham. Sprinkle with cloves. Place in shallow baking pan. Bake at 350° F for 20 minutes. Arrange figs and bananas in pan around ham. Brush with combination of maple syrup, lemon juice and bananas. Heat an additional 15 minutes; brush again with sauce. Makes 4 to 5 servings.

### Fig & Sun-Dried Tomato Pizza

*You can put together this trendy, and very flavorful pizza almost as quickly as calling for delivery. California figs add a surprising richness and complement the robust onion and garlic.*

2 tablespoons olive oil
¼ cup chopped fresh basil, oregano
(or Italian parsley)
1 medium sweet or red onion, sliced
2 to 4 cloves garlic, minced
1 cup shredded part-skim Mozzarella,

Provolone or Monterey Jack cheese
1 cup California figs, sliced, stems removed
1 (12 to 14-inch) prepared pizza crust or
pizza bread base
¼ cup sun-dried tomatoes, chopped
2 tablespoons balsamic vinegar

Heat oil in large skillet. Add onion, garlic, figs and tomatoes and cook until onions are just tender. Stir in balsamic vinegar and basil. Sprinkle Mozzarella evenly over pizza crust and top with fig mixture. Bake in preheated 425° F oven until crust is browned, about 10 to 15 minutes. Cut wedges to serve. Makes 1 (14-inch) pizza, about 8 servings.

### Seared Cod with Fig Tapenade

1 cup calamata olives, pitted and finely chopped
8 dried figs, finely chopped
2 Tbsp capers, finely chopped
2 Tbsp finely chopped basil, plus 4 leaves
for garnish
½ cup, plus 2 Tbsp extra virgin olive oil
Ground pepper
4 to 6 oz. cod fillets
Salt

Directions: In a bowl, combine the olives with the figs, capers, chopped basil and olive oil. Season with pepper. Preheat oven to 360° F. In a heavy skillet, heat 1 tablespoon olive oil. Season the fish with salt and pepper. Add 2 of the fillets to the skillet. Cook over high heat until browned on the bottom, about 3 minutes. Turn and cook just until opaque throughout, about 3 minutes. Remove fish. Keep it warm in the oven. Repeat with the remaining 1 tablespoon olive oil and cod fillets. Transfer the fish to dinner plates and spoon the tapenade over the top. Garnish with the basil leaves and serve.

### Fig & Wild Rice Chicken Salad

½ cup long-grain brown rice
¼ teaspoon *each* grated lemon peel and pepper
½ cup wild rice
¾ cup plain nonfat yogurt
2 cups shredded cooked chicken
½ cup sliced green onion
½ cup chopped pecans, toasted
3 tablespoons olive oil
8 oz Blue Ribbon Orchard Choice or Sun-Maid Calimyrna or Mission Figs
1 1/2-2 tablespoons lemon juice
1 teaspoon salt

In medium saucepan, bring 2¼ cups water to a boil. Add brown and wild rice. Cover and reduce heat to low; cook 55 minutes until water is absorbed and rice is done. Cool. Remove stems from figs and quarter. In large bowl, combine yogurt and next six ingredients. Stir in rice, chicken, pecans and figs. Refrigerate until serving. Makes 6 servings.

### Figs Clafouti

½ cup part-skim or nonfat ricotta cheese
4 large eggs, lightly beaten
1½ cups buttermilk
2 tsp grated lemon zest
1 cup unbleached all-purpose flour
1 tsp vanilla extract
2 Tbsp sugar
8 tender ripe figs, stem removed and sliced

Directions: Place the ricotta in the work bowl of a food processor or blender and process until smooth. Add the buttermilk. Process again to blend. Add the flour, sugar, eggs, lemon zest and vanilla. Process to make a smooth batter. Transfer to a larger bowl. Cover with plastic wrap. Lightly grease an 8-inch baking dish or six individual ramekins with unsalted butter or vegetable oil. Place the pared figs at the bottom of the dish and pour the batter evenly on top.

*Sprinkle figs with ¼ cup brown sugar before putting them into the baking dish.
Place the dishes inside a large baking dish and add water to the outer dish until it comes halfway up the side of the clafouti. Bake until puffy and golden, about 40 minutes. Checking occasionally, add water as necessary to maintain the level. If the top starts browning too quickly, cover loosely with foil.

### California Fig & Goat Cheese Pizza

1 tablespoon *each* of butter and olive oil
1 tablespoon chopped fresh thyme or
1 teaspoon dried
3 large onions (1½ lbs.), thinly sliced
1 tablespoon balsamic or red wine vinegar
1 12-inch Italian bread shell or pizza crust
½ teaspoon salt
¼ teaspoon pepper
2/3 cup (3½ oz.) crumbled mild goat cheese
1 cup thinly sliced Blue Ribbon Orchard Choice or Sun-Maid Mission or Calimyrna Figs

Heat oven to 450° F. In large deep skillet or Dutch oven, melt butter in oil over medium heat. Stir in onions, vinegar, salt and pepper; cook, stirring occasionally, until softened and golden brown, 25-30 minutes. Stir in figs and thyme; remove from heat. (Onion-fig mixture can be made ahead and refrigerated.) Spread onion-fig mixture evenly over pizza crust and top with cheese. Bake until crust is crisp and cheese has softened, 8-10 minutes.
Makes 8 servings.

### Roasted Salmon with Caramelized Onions, Figs & Wine

2 tablespoons olive oil
1 tablespoon balsamic vinegar
1 pound yellow onions, halved and thinly sliced to measure 4 cups
1 tablespoon chopped fresh rosemary
1 teaspoon dried rosemary
Salt
Freshly ground black pepper
Chopped parsley
1 cup (6 oz.) Blue ribbon Orchard Choice or Sun-Maid Mission or Calimyrna Figs
1 to 1 ⅓ pounds salmon filet, skinned and cut into 4 portions
½ cup red or white wine
½ cup chicken broth

Swirl olive oil in bottom of medium nonstick skillet. Add onions and sprinkle with ½ teaspoon

*Roasted Salmon*

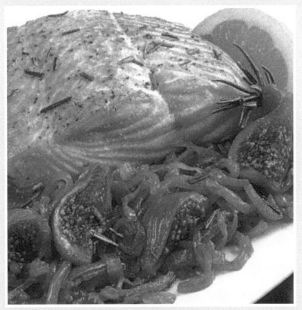

salt. Cover and cook over medium-low heat, stirring occasionally, until onions are soft, about 10 minutes. Remove cover and cook, stirring often, until onions are golden, 15 to 20 minutes. Cut stems from figs and halve. Stir in figs, wine, broth, vinegar and fresh rosemary. Increase heat to high and simmer until sauce thickens, about 5 minutes. Add salt and pepper to taste. Keep warm. Preheat oven to 450° F. Sprinkle salmon with salt and pepper to taste. Place on lightly oiled heavy baking sheet. Roast for 7 to 10 minutes or until fish flakes. Sprinkle salmon with parsley. Serve over fig sauce. Makes 4 servings.

### Western Wheat Pilaf

½ cup finely chopped onion
Sherry
2 tablespoons margarine
½ cup finely chopped California Dried Figs
1 cup bulgur wheat
2 chicken-flavored bouillon cubes
3 tablespoons sesame seeds or pine nuts
2 cups water
Juice of one orange (about ¼ cup)
1 teaspoon finely grated orange peel

Sauté onion in margarine until soft. Stir in wheat to coat with margarine. Add low fat chicken bouillon cubes and water. Measure orange juice and add enough sherry to make ½ cup. Add to pilaf. Cover and simmer over low heat for 35 minutes. Five minutes before serving, stir in figs, sesame seeds or pine nuts and orange peel. Cover to complete cooking. Makes 4 to 6 servings.

### Fig-Chicken Crunch Sandwich Spread

2 (4-¾ ounce) cans chicken spread
1 (3 ounce) package cream cheese
½ cup chopped California Dried Figs
¼ cup finely chopped nuts
1 teaspoon minced candied ginger

Combine chicken spread with cream cheese, California dried figs, nuts and ginger. Use as a sandwich filling. Makes about 2 cups.

### Fig & Walnut Pasta with Gorgonzola

2 tablespoons butter
½ cup chopped walnuts
1 large onion, sliced
½ teaspoon salt
8 ounces vermicelli or linguine
1½ cups (6 oz.) crumbed Gorgonzola cheese
2 tablespoons olive oil
1 cup (6 oz.) Blue Ribbon Orchard Choice or Sun-Maid Calimyrna or Mission Figs

Heat butter in large skillet. Add onion and sauté over medium-high heat 10-12 minutes, stirring frequently, until golden brown. Meanwhile prepare pasta according to package directions. Drain; toss with olive oil and set aside. Remove stems from figs and coarsely chop. Stir figs, walnuts and salt into onions; cook 2 minutes or until heated through. Pour mixture over pasta. Sprinkle with Gorgonzola and toss gently. Serve immediately. Makes 4-6 servings.

### Pork Medallions with Honey-Glazed Figs & Apples

2 tart green apples, about 1 pound
2 teaspoons vegetable oil
1 cup Blue Ribbon Orchard Choice or Sun Maid Mission or Calimyrna Figs
½ cup white wine or water

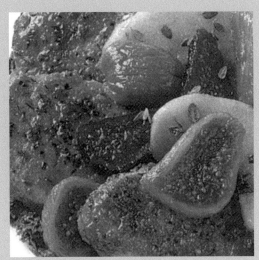
*Pork Medallions with Honey-Glazed Figs and Apples*

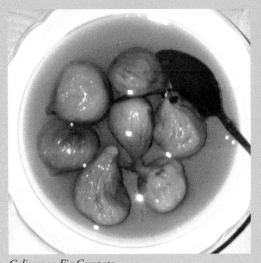
*Calimyrna Fig Compote*

3 tablespoons honey
1 pound pork tenderloin
Parsley or fresh thyme for garnish
*Thyme Seasoning, recipe follows*

Peel and core apples; cut each into 16 wedges. Remove stems and halve figs. Cut tenderloin into ¾-inch thick slices; rub with thyme seasoning. Heal oil in medium frying pan over medium-high heat; add pork and cook 2 minutes on each side. Reduce heat and cook until firm, about 3 to 4 minutes. Remove and keep warm. Stir apples, figs and wine into pan. Simmer until liquid evaporates, about 8 minutes. Add honey; stir until apples are tender and glazed, about 2 minutes. Pour fig mixture over pork and garnish with parsley or thyme. Makes 4 servings.

Thyme Seasoning: Stir together 1 tablespoon vegetable oil, 1 tablespoon onion powder, 1¾ teaspoons thyme leaves, 1 teaspoon salt and 1 teaspoon ground black pepper.

## DESSERT FIGS

### *Figs Compote*

8 to 10 small dried figs
1 cup water
1/8 tsp cardamom, ground

Directions: Wash dried figs carefully. Soak figs into bowl with one cup water; warm water is best. Soak overnight. Serve early morning.

### *Fig Stuffed with Orange-Anise Cream*

16 dried figs
2 tsp grated orange rind
4 oz nonfat cream cheese
1½ tsp honey
1 Tbsp fresh orange juice
½ tsp aniseed, crushed

Directions: Trim and discard the stems from the figs. Cut down through the stem end vertically and horizontally to make an X. Gently push each fig open. Place the figs on a platter, cut side up. In a medium bowl, combine the cream cheese, orange juice, orange rind, honey and aniseed. With electric beaters or a wooden spoon, beat until creamy. Spoon a dollop of the mixture into the center of each fig. Serve immediately or cover with plastic wrap and refrigerate for two hours.

## Fig Maple Pudding

¼ lb figs
¼ tsp salt
¾ cup maple syrup
1½ tsp sugar
½ cup boiling water
3 Tbsp shortening
¾ cup sifted flour
¼ to 1/3 cup milk
1½ tsp baking powder

Directions: Soften figs in cold water. Cut into halves. Place in greased baking dish. Mix maple syrup with boiling water, pour over figs. Cover dish and steam for ½ hour. Sift flour, baking powder, salt and sugar together. Cut in shortening with two knives or pastry blender. Add milk and mix lightly. Remove baking dish from steamer and pour batter over figs. Cover dish. Return to steamer and steam one hour. This pudding provides its own sauce.

## Ricotta-Filled Figs

2 Tbsp red wine
2 Tbsp pine nuts
1 whole cinnamon stick
1 cup ricotta cheese
1 2-inch slice lemon peel, yellow part only
1 Tbsp honey
8 large dried mission figs
1 tsp grated lemon zest

Directions: Put the wine, cinnamon stick and lemon peel in a medium saucepan and add two cups water. Cover and bring to a boil over medium-high heat. Reduce heat to medium-low and simmer 15 minutes to allow the cinnamon and lemon to steep. Add the figs and bring back to a gentle simmer uncovered over medium heat. Remove from heat, cover and let sit until the figs have softened, about 40 minutes. Drain and let cool. Spread the pine nuts in a single layer on a sheet of aluminum foil on a toaster tray. Place in the toaster oven and toast on "light" setting, watching carefully to make sure they don't burn. Remove from the oven when golden brown, about 2 minutes. In a small mixing bowl, combine the ricotta, honey, lemon zest and pine nuts. Carefully slice off the top (stem end) of each fig. Using a teaspoon, stuff as much filling into the center of each fig without forcing it to split. Refrigerate until chilled through, about 3 hours.

*Chunky Fig Bread*

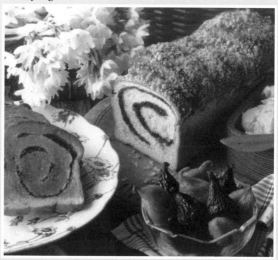

## Fig Banana Brick

2 Tbsp quick-cooking tapioca
1 cup dried figs
1½ cups milk
1 cup mashed bananas
2 Tbsp sugar
½ tsp grated lemon rind
1/8 tsp salt
2 tsp vanilla

Directions: Cook tapioca and milk over hot water about 10 minutes. Strain but do not rub tapioca through the sieve. Add sugar and salt to strained milk mixture. Chill. Boil figs 10 minutes in water to cover. Drain and cool. Clip stems and chop. Whip cream until stiff. Combine with figs, cold milk mixture, bananas, lemon rind and vanilla. Mix thoroughly. Pour into freezing tray of refrigerator and freeze. Stirring 2 to 3 times. Unmold and slice.

## Fig Bread

½ cup raisins
½ Tbsp salt
½ cup figs
1 tsp baking soda
2 Tbsp shortening
1 tsp baking powder
1 cup honey
¾ cup milk
1 egg
¼ cup sour milk
2½ cups sifted flour
1 cup nuts

Directions: Cut raisins and figs into small pieces. Cream shortening with honey until fluffy. Add beaten egg. Sift dry ingredients together. Add alternately with milk. Add nuts and fruits. Bake in moderate oven 325° F for one 1¼ hours.

## Breakfast Figs

6 quarts fresh figs
1 gallon boiling water
1 cup baking soda
6 cups water
6 cups honey
1 lemon or orange, optional

Directions: Select figs of uniform size and ripeness. Add soda to boiling water and pour into unpeeled figs. Let stand 5 to 10 minutes. When skins become slightly transparent, remove to a bath of cold water and rinse thoroughly. Combine honey and water. Heat to boiling. Add figs and simmer until figs can be pierced with a straw and the skins cook clear and translucent. Pack in sterile jars. Fill with hot syrup. One sliced lemon and one sliced orange may be added to each jar. Adjust rings and cover. Process 25 minutes in hot water bath.

## Fig Cake

1 cup buttermilk
1 tsp cinnamon
1 cup oil
1 tsp vanilla
3 eggs
1 tsp allspice
1½ cups flour
1 cup chopped nuts
1 tsp baking soda
1 cup preserves
1 tsp salt

Glaze: ½ cup buttermilk
1 cup sugar
¾ stick butter
½ tsp baking soda

Directions: Combine all of the cake ingredients. Bake in a bundt pan at 375° for one hour. Glaze ingredients can cook until the soft ball stage. Pour on the warm cake.

## Fig-Walnut Loaf

2 cups sifted flour
1 cup toasted English walnuts, coarsely chopped
1 tsp salt
½ cup dried figs, chopped fine
4 tsp baking powder
1 egg
1/3 cup sugar
1½ cups milk
1 cup whole-wheat flour

Directions: Sift first four ingredients together.
Mix in whole-wheat flour, nuts and figs. Beat
egg slightly and add milk. Add liquid to dry
ingredients, stirring only enough to dampen
all the flour. Pour into greased loaf pan. Bake
in moderate oven (350° F) one hour.

## Fig Cookies

2¼ cups sifted cake flour
2 eggs, beaten
½ tsp cinnamon
2 Tbsp sour cream
½ cup shortening
1 cup chopped figs
1 cup brown sugar
1 tsp soda

Directions: Sift flour, cinnamon and soda together.
Cream shortening with sugar until fluffy. Add eggs,
sour cream and figs. Add sifted dry ingredients
with more flour if necessary. Chill thoroughly. Roll
out on lightly floured board to 1/8 inch thickness.
Cut with cookie cutter and bake on greased
cookie sheet in moderate oven (350° F) for 10
to 12 minutes or until browned.

## Fig Refrigerator Cake

1 cup cooked dried figs
2 eggs, separated with salt
1½ tsp unflavored gelatin
1 tsp vanilla
1 Tbsp cold water
½ cup heavy whipped cream
1¼ cup milk
12 marshmallows, quartered
4 Tbsp sugar
Graham crackers

Directions: Clip stems from figs and cut figs into
pieces. Soften gelatin in cold water. Scald 1-cup
milk over hot water. Caramelize two tablespoons
sugar and dissolve in hot water. Combine egg
yolks, ¼ cup cold milk, remaining sugar and salt.
Stir into hot milk. Continue cooking until custard
coats the spoon. Add figs and gelatin. Cool. Add
flavoring, stiffly beaten egg whites filling slightly
over ½ full. Cover. Steam for 45 minutes. Serve
hot with lemon, vanilla or marshmallow sauce.
They maybe reheated.

## Maple Fig Cake

1 cup dried figs
1 cup sugar
2¾ cups sifted flour
2 eggs, well beaten
1 tsp salt
¾ cup milk
3 tsp baking powder
½ tsp maple flavoring
¾ cup shortening

Directions: Pour boiling water over figs. Cover.
Let stand for five minutes. Drain, dry on a towel.

Clip stems and slice fine. Sift flour, salt and baking powder together. Cream shortening with sugar until fluffy. Add eggs. Beat thoroughly. Add sifted dry ingredients and milk alternately in small amounts, beating well after each addition. Add flavoring and figs and mix lightly but thoroughly. Pour into greased pan. Bake in moderate oven (350° F) for one hour and 20 minutes.

### Apple-Fig Crumble
This crumble made with dried figs is an ideal Fall dessert.

1 bottle Madeira
1 vanilla bean, split lengthwise
1½ cups sugar
8 granny smith apples, peeled, cored and sliced
15 dried figs, chopped
4 cups streusel topping
3 sticks of cinnamon
1½ cups of crème Anglaise (Vanilla custard sauce)

Directions: Preheat oven to 350° F. Lightly coat eight 3"x1½" ramekins with vegetable cooking spray. In a medium saucepan bring the Madeira, sugar, figs, cinnamon sticks and vanilla to a boil. Reduce heat to medium and cook for 20 to 30 minutes until thickened and reduced by half. Place apples in a medium ovenproof bowl. Remove the saucepan from the heat and pour into mixture over apples. Stir the mixture until well combined. Let cool. Discard the vanilla bean. Evenly divide the apple-fig mixture among the prepared ramekins. Top each with ½ cup of streusel topping. Place the ramekins on a baking sheet and bake for 25 to 30 minutes until the top is golden and the mixture starts to bubble. Serve with crème Anglaise or if desired, a high-quality purchased vanilla ice cream.

### Fig Pudding

¾ cup chopped figs
½ tsp baking soda
¾ cup shortening
1 tsp cinnamon
1 cup sugar
½ cup sour milk
2 eggs
1 tsp vanilla
2 cups sifted flour

Directions: Rinse figs and dry on a towel. Clip stems and force enough through food chopper to measure ¾ cup. Cream shortening and sugar together until fluffy. Add beaten eggs. Mix. Add figs and blend well. Sift flour, salt, soda and spice together. Add alternately with milk in small amounts, mixing well after each addition. Stir in flavoring. Pour into greased custard cups, filling slightly over ½ full. Cover. Steam for 45 minutes. Serve hot with lemon, vanilla or marshmallow sauce. They may be reheated.

### Fig Parfait
½ cup dried chopped figs
¼ cup water
¼ cup light brown sugar
1 pint vanilla ice cream
½ cup chopped walnuts
Whipped cream

Directions: Cook chopped figs, sugar and water until slightly thickened. Add nut meats and chill. Arrange alternate layers of ice cream and chilled fig sauce in parfait glasses. Top with whipped cream.

### Fig Konfyt

2 lb green unripe figs
4 cups granulated sugar
4 tsp salt
½ cup water
1 tsp baking soda

Directions: Trim the stem off each fig, then with a small sharp knife cut a deep cross into the top. Place the figs in a large glass bowl. Cover with cold water and add the salt. Mix well until the salt is dissolved, then weigh down with a plate and let stand overnight. The next day, bring a large pan of water to a boil with the baking soda. Drain the figs and add the salt. Mix well until the salt is dissolved, then weigh down with a plate and let stand overnight. Return to a boil, then reduce the heat and simmer gently for 25-30 minutes or until the figs are just tender. Have ready a large bowl of very cold water and immediately transfer the figs to it. Let cool, then drain the figs well. Place in a large non-corrosive saucepan. Place the sugar and water in a separate pan. Bring to a boil, stirring until the sugar is dissolved, then skim well. Boil for 5 minutes then pour over the figs. Weigh down and stand overnight. The next day, bring slowly to a boil and then simmer very gently for 2 to 2½ hours. Lift them out of the syrup with a slotted spoon and arrange in the hot sterilized jars.

### Fig Roll

2 cups sifted flour
1 cup sugar
1½ tsp baking powder
4 Tbsp cold water
¾ tsp salt

1 tsp vanilla
6 eggs, separated

Directions: Sift flour, baking powder and salt together four times. Beat egg yokes very thoroughly. Add sugar. Beat until thick enough to hold a soft peak. Add water and flavoring, folding softest dry ingredients in small amounts. Beat egg whites until stiff, but not dry. Fold into batter. Pour into shallow pan. Line with paper. Bake in moderate oven (350° F) 12 to 15 minutes. Turn out onto towel, cut off crusts. Unroll and spread with fig filling. Roll. Top may be spread with vanilla cream frosting.

### Fig Turnover

1 cup sugar
1/3 cup lemon juice
1 Tbsp flour
2 Tbsp grated lemon rind
½ cup water and fig juice
1 cup canned figs chopped
1 Tbsp butter
1 recipe plain pastry
1 egg, beaten

Directions: Combine first 8 ingredients. Cook slowly until thickened. Cool. Roll pastry 1/8 inch thick. Cut into 4 inch circles. Place a tablespoon of fig mixture on half of each circle. Moisten edges. Fold other half over filling. Pinch edges together. Prick top. Place on baking sheet. Bake in very hot oven (450° F) about 15 minutes.

### Three-Citrus Custard with Fresh Figs

1 cup lemon juice
¼ lb unsalted butter, cut into small pieces

½ cup grapefruit juice
1 Tbsp finely grated lemon zest
½ cup orange juice
1 Tbsp finely grated orange zest
6 large eggs
8 figs, preferably green & purple, cut into
thick wedges
1 cup sugar
Butter cookie for serving

Directions: In a double boiler, in a large heat proof bowl, set over a saucepan filled with about one inch of simmer water. Whisk the citrus juices with the eggs and sugar until combined. Cook, stirring constantly with a wooden spoon until the custard is smooth and thick, 10-20 minutes. Do not boil. Remove the custard from the heat. Stir in butter. Strain the custard into bowl. Stir in the grated citrus zests. Stir for one minute to cool slightly, then cover with waxed paper or plastic. Refrigerate overnight. Spoon the custard into shallow bowl of stemmed glasses. Garnish with the zests.

### Fig Melba

3 medium to large ripe figs
½ cup raspberry puree
½ pint fresh raspberries
Fancy garnishing cookies
6 large scoops vanilla bean ice cream

Directions: Quarter figs. Pick fresh figs through the berries. Place a scoop of ice cream in a glass bowl. Pour raspberry puree over the ice cream. Surround with slices of figs and a few fresh raspberries. Garnish with fancy cookies, if desired.

### Baked Figs with Honey Ice Cream

1½ cups half and half cream
1 Tbsp unsalted butter, cut into small pieces
1½ cups heavy cream
12 large or 18 small ripe figs, halved lengthwise
6 eggs
1 Tbsp sugar
½ cup, plus 2 Tbsp honey

To make the ice cream: Place saucepan over medium heat. Combine the half and half cream and the heavy cream. Heat until almost boiling. While the cream heats, in a large bowl whisk the egg yolks and honey until smooth. Gradually whisk in half of the hot cream, then return the mixture to the saucepan. Cook over medium heat stirring constantly until the mixture visibly thickens and forms a custard, about 3 minutes. Do not let it boil. Let cool. Refrigerate to chill thoroughly. Freeze the custard in an ice-cream maker according to the manufacturer's directions. Store in freezer until needed.

To bake the figs: Preheat oven to 425° F. Choose a baking sheet large enough to hold the halved figs in a single layer. Dot the bottom of the dish with the butter. Arrange the figs in the prepared dish. Cut side up and sprinkle with sugar. Bake until bubbling hot and tender, about 15 minutes. Divide half of the figs among dessert goblets, balloon wine glasses or compote dish. Top each serving with some of the ice cream or the remaining figs and any syrupy juices in the baking dish. You will have ice cream left over, serve immediately.

### Fresh Figs and Plums in Manzanill
Manzanilla is a very dry, pale sherry, used here as the basis of a syrup in which the figs and the plums are macerate.

1 cup Manzanilla or other dry sherry
6 plums, pitted and quartered
2 imported bay leaves
¼ cup crème fraiche
½ tsp minced lemon zest
3 Tbsp sugar
8 fresh black figs, stemmed and quartered

Directions: In a medium saucepan, cook the sherry with the sugar, bay leaves and lemon zest over moderately high heat, stirring just until the sugar dissolves. Transfer the mixture to a large bowl. Let cool. Add figs and plums. Let stand for 15 minutes. Toss occasionally. Discard the bay leaves. Serve the fruit in shallow bowls topped with a dollop of crème fraiche. Serve with biscotti.

### Figs with Honey and Champagne
Good luck ingredients—figs, honey and bay leaves. It is good with an indulgent sweet for a cold winter day.

1 lb dried calimyrna figs
2 tsp sugar
1 cup warm water
3 long strips lemon zest
1½ cups dry sparkling wine
3 bay leaves
1 tsp honey
½ tsp fennel seeds, lightly toasted

Directions: In medium saucepan combine the figs and water and let stand for one hour. Add the sparkling wine, honey, sugar, lemon zest and bay leaves. Bring to boil. Reduce heat to low. Simmer the figs until they are softened, about 20 minutes. With a slotted spoon, transfer the softened figs to a bowl. Boil the cooking liquid until it is syrupy, about 6 to 8 minutes. Remove the strips of lemon

zest and the bay leaves from the syrup. Pour the syrup over the figs. Sprinkle the figs with the fennel seeds and serve warm.

### Fig Moon

1½ cups flour
1/3 cup light-brown sugar
½ tsp baking powder
1 large egg
½ tsp baking soda
½ tsp finely grated lemon zest
¼ tsp cinnamon
8 medium dried figs, stemmed and quartered
¼ tsp salt
½ cup pitted dates
4 Tbsp unsalted butter
1/3 cup water
¼ cup vegetable shortening
2 tsp cognac or water

Directions: In a medium bowl stir the flour with the baking powder, baking soda, cinnamon and salt. In a large bowl using an electric mixer, cream the butter and shortening with the brown sugar until fluffy. Beat in the egg and zest. Using a wooden spoon stir in the dry ingredients. Shape into a disk, wrap in waxed paper and refrigerate until firm, at least 3 hours or overnight. In a small non-reactive saucepan combine the figs, dates and water. Bring to simmer over moderate heat and cook until the figs are tender, about 12 minutes. Transfer the fruit and its cooking liquid to food processor. Add the cognac and puree until smooth. Let cool completely.

Heat the oven to 375° F. Cut the chilled dough into quarters. On a lightly floured work surface roll out one piece of the dough 1/8-inch thick.

Cut with a 3-inch fluted round cookie cutter. Arrange the rounds about one inch apart on a large cookie sheet. Continue rolling and cutting the dough until the cookie sheet is full. Knead the scraps together and refrigerate until chilled. Spoon one teaspoon of the fig filling into the center of each round. Fold the dough over the filling to form a half moon. Press the edges with the tines of a fork to seal. Using a small sharp knife cut two vents in the top of each cookie. Bake until golden and set, about 12 minutes. Cool completely. Continue making cookies with the remaining dough, scraps and filling.

### Citrus Custard Tarts with Caramelized Figs

½ cup lemon juice
4 Tbsp unsalted butter, cut into pieces
¼ cup grapefruit juice
½ Tbsp finely grated lemon zest
¼ cup orange juice
½ Tbsp finely grated orange zest
3 large eggs
12 ripe fresh figs, preferably green and purple, cut into wedges
1 cup sugar
½ cup water
Tart shells

Directions: In a double boiler or heatproof bowl, set over a saucepan filled with about an inch of simmering water. Whisk the citrus juices together with the eggs and ½ cup of the sugar until blended. Cook, stirring constantly with a wooden spoon, until the custard is smooth and thick, 10 to 12 minutes. Do not boil. Remove from heat. Stir in butter. Strain custard into a bowl and stir in the citrus zests. Divide the custard among the tart shells. Let cool completely. Cover with a sheet of waxed paper and refrigerate overnight. Remove the tarts from the pans and arrange the figs on top. In a small saucepan, cook the remaining ½ cup sugar with the water over moderate heat, stirring occasionally until the sugar is dissolved and syrup slightly thickened, about 5 minutes. Let the syrup cook, then brush over the figs to glaze.

### Tart Shells

2½ cups flour
½ lb cold unsalted butter, cut into ½ pieces
2 tsp sugar
1 tsp finely grated lemon zest
¾ tsp salt
¼ cup plus 3 Tbsp cold skim milk

Directions: In a food processor, combine the flour, sugar and salt and pulse to blend. Add butter and lemon zest and pulse until the mixture resembles course meal. Add milk and pulse just until combined. Transfer the dough to a lightly floured work surface and gently knead until smooth. Divide the dough in half and pat each half into a smooth disk. Wrap in plastic and refrigerate until the dough is chilled. Arrange eight 41/2 inch fluted tart pans with removable bottoms on a baking sheet. Divide one disk of dough into four equal pieces and roll each piece out to a 61/2 inch round. Press each round into a tart pan against the sides. Trim the pastry even with the rims of the pan. Refrigerate the tart shells for 30 minutes. Heat the oven to 375° F. Line each shell with a piece of foil and fill with pie weight, dried beans or rice. Bake until the edges are lightly golden, about 25 minutes. Remove the foil and weights. Bake until the pastry bottoms are golden, about 7 minutes longer. Let cool before filling.

### Hot Fruit Appetizer

9 slices bacon
Some Roquefort cheese
12 fresh figs
Some Cream cheese
12 unpitted dates
slices of ham

Directions: Cut bacon into pieces long enough to wrap one time around the figs and dates. Remove hard stem end of figs and make a gash on sides with a sharp paring knife. Mix together equal quantities of Roquefort and cream cheese and fill the figs. Wrap in bacon and secure with a wooden pick. Pit dates and fill with equal quantities of cream cheese and ham. Wrap in bacon too. Thread the figs and dates on a long skewer and broil, turning several times until the bacon is crisp. Serve hot from the skewer or keep hot in a small, covered dish.

### Cookies
Use your favorite cookie recipe and fill with one of these special fig fillings:

### Poached Fig Topping
1½ cups dried figs
3 Tbsp sugar
2 cups water
2 Tbsp lemon juice
½ cup bourbon

Directions: In a saucepan simmer figs, water, bourbon, sugar and lemon juice for 10 minutes. Cool figs syrup to room temperature.

### Fig Filling

1 cup sugar
¼ tsp salt
2 Tbsp butter
4 cups chopped figs
1-1/3 cups hot water

### Fig-Lemon Filling

1½ cups water
¼ Tbsp salt
1 cup sugar
2 cups chopped figs
4 Tbsp flour
Juice of two lemons

### Fig-Orange Filling

1 cup water
3 cups chopped figs
1 cup sugar
½ cup orange juice
¼ tsp salt
4 tsp grated orange rind
1 cup chopped nuts

### Walnut Fig Filling

1¼ cups water
¾ cups chopped walnuts
1 cup corn syrup
2 cups chopped figs
½ cup sugar
2 Tbsp lemon juice
4 Tbsp flour
2 tsp grated lemon rind
¼ tsp salt

## Fig Heavenly Sauce

2 egg yolks
1/3 cup slivered toasted almonds
1 cup powdered sugar
2/3 cup chopped California dried figs
1 cup heavy cream, whipped
½ teaspoon finely chopped candied ginger

Beat egg yolks with powdered sugar until smooth and thick; fold into whipped cream. Gently fold in nuts, dried figs and ginger. Spoon over ice cream, chiffon cake or fruits. Makes 6 servings.

## Fig Aloha Cookies

1/3 cup butter or margarine
1/8 teaspoon salt
½ cup sugar
1 (8 ounce) can crushed pineapple, drained
1 egg
¼ cup chopped macadamia nuts or walnuts
1 ½ cups sifted flour
½ cup chopped California dried figs
¼ teaspoon baking soda

Glaze: : 1 cup powdered sugar
2 tablespoons milk
Flaked coconut

In large bowl, beat butter, sugar and egg until fluffy. Combine flour, soda and salt; beat into butter-sugar mixture alternately with pineapple. Stir in nuts and figs. Drop by teaspoon on greased cookie sheet. Bake at 350° F for 10 to 12 minutes. While warm, dip cookies into glaze of powdered sugar and milk; then in coconut. Makes about 3 dozen.

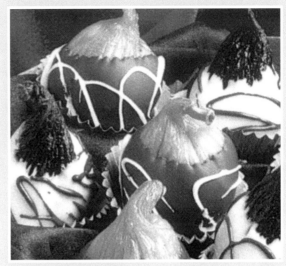

*Chocolate-Dipped Stuffed Figs*

## California Figs Confection

½ cup margarine
1 can (14 oz.) non-fat sweetened condensed milk
1 cup graham cracker crumbs  (about 18 squares)
½ cup coconut (flaked shredded, unsweetened)
½ cup *each* wheat germ and sunflower seeds
1 cup chopped California Dried Figs
1 cup chopped walnuts

Melt margarine in a 9x13-inch baking pan—either in microwave or in pre-heating oven. Mix in cracker crumbs, wheat germ, sunflower seeds, and figs; press in an even layer. Pour non-fat sweetened condensed milk evenly over crumb mixture. Top with coconut and walnuts, pressing down lightly. Bake in a 350° F oven for 25 to 30 minutes until toasty brown. Cool. Serve from pan in small squares or break into toffee-like pieces. Enjoy like candy, or trail mix, or top fresh fruit or ice cream with melt-in-your-mouth California Fig Confection.

### Chocolate-Dipped Stuffed Figs

15 Blue Ribbon Orchard Choice or
Sun-Maid Mission or Calimyrna Figs
15 to 30 small pieces candied ginger, toasted nuts
(walnuts, pecans, hazelnuts, almonds or
macadamias) or chocolate
¾ cup sugar
¾ cup water
1/2 cup brandy (or 1/2 cup water mixed with
1 1/2 teaspoons vanilla extract)
5 to 6 ounces semisweet,
bittersweets or premium white chocolate, chopped

With sharp knife, cut small slit in bottom of each
fig. In small saucepan, heat sugar and water over
medium heat until sugar dissolves. Stir in brandy
and figs. Bring to a boil over high heat then reduce
heat and simmer 20 minutes. Drain figs, cool and
dry thoroughly. Stuff one or two pieces of ginger,
nuts and/or chocolate into each fig. Place chopped
chocolate in 1-cup glass measuring cup or small
microwave-safe bowl. Heat on medium/50%
power until almost melted, stirring after every 1 to
1½ minutes. Remove from oven and stir until
melted. Hold stem of each fig and dip in melted
chocolate. Place figs, stems up, in wax paper-lined
tray until chocolate sets. Store in airtight container
in refrigerator. Makes 15 figs.

### Chocolate-Fig Pecan Bars

2 cups all-purpose flour
¾ cup chopped pecans
¾ cup sugar, divided
2/3 cup semisweet chocolate pieces
10 tablespoons butter or margarine
3 large eggs
8 ounces Blue Ribbon Orchard Choice or
Sun-Maid Mission or Calimyrna Figs
¾ cup light corn syrup
1 teaspoon vanilla extract

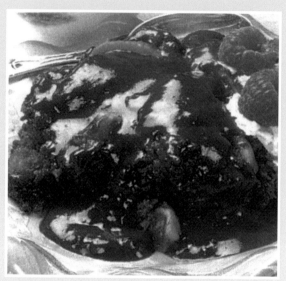
*Figgy Fudgy Pudding Cake*

Heat oven to 350° F. Stir together flour and ¼ cup
sugar. Add butter. With pastry blender or 2 knives,
cut butter into dry ingredients until mixture
resembles course crumbs. (Mixture will be dry.)
Press in bottom of lightly greased 13 x 9-inch
baking pan. Bake for 15 minutes or until edges
begin to brown. Remove stems from figs and
chop. Sprinkle figs, pecans and chocolate pieces
over crust. Lightly beat eggs, gradually beat in
remaining ½ cup sugar, corn syrup and vanilla
until well blended. Pour over crust. Return to oven
for 20 to 30 minutes or until filling is firm around
edges and slightly soft at center. Cool on wire rack.
Makes 32 bars.

### Deep Dish Pear Cobbler with Lemon Infused Figs

8 ounces Blue Ribbon Orchard Choice or
Sun-Maid Mission or Calimyrna Figs
2 pounds firm, ripe pears, peeled and
sliced (about ½-inch thick)
1/3 cup *each* granulated and packed brown sugar
3 tablespoons lemon juice

¾ teaspoon finely grated lemon peel
1 teaspoon ground cinnamon
2 tablespoons cornstarch mixed with 2
tablespoons water
Prepared refrigerated or frozen pastry for
9-inch pie or 1 sheet frozen puff pastry

Topping:
1 tablespoon granulated sugar,
1/3 cup chopped walnuts

Remove stems from figs and slice. In large
saucepan, combine figs, sugars, lemon juice and
peel, cinnamon and 2 tablespoons water. Bring to
boil over medium-high heat and stir to dissolve
sugar. Stir in cornstarch mixture and cook until
slightly thickened. Remove from heat and stir in
pears. Turn into 2-quart baking dish such as 8-inch
square baking pan or 9 x 2-inch round cake pan.
Bring pastry to room temperature according to
package directions. With 2½ to 3-inch cookie
or biscuit cutter, cut pastry into 9 to 12 pieces.
Arrange pastry, slightly over-lapping, on filling.
Sprinkle with topping ingredients. Bake in
preheated 400°F oven for 20 to 25 minutes or
until filling is bubbly and crust is golden. Serve
warm or at room temperature, with vanilla ice
cream, if desired. Makes 6 to 8 servings.

*Fabulous Fig Bars*

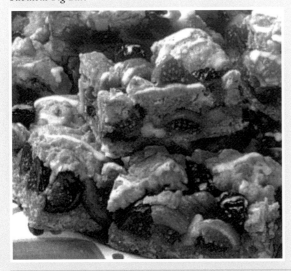

## Figgy Fudgy Pudding Cake

1 cup all-purpose flour
1/3 cup semisweet chocolate pieces, optional
2/3 cup sugar
¼ cup chopped, toasted pecans
¼ teaspoon salt
¾ cup packed light brown sugar
½ cup milk
¼ cup unsweetened cocoa powder
¼ cup butter, melted
1¾ cups hottest tap water
1½ teaspoons vanilla extract
1 cup chopped Blue Ribbon Orchard
Choice or Sun-Maid Mission or Calimyrna
Figs, stems removed

Heat oven to 350° F. In ungreased 8 or 9-inch
square pan, stir together flour, sugar, 3 tablespoons
cocoa powder, baking powder and salt. With fork,
blend in milk, butter and vanilla until smooth. Stir
in figs, chocolate pieces and pecans. Sprinkle
brown sugar and remaining ¼ cup cocoa evenly
over top. Pour hot water evenly over top. Do not
stir. Bake for 35 to 40 minutes, until sauce forms
on bottom and cake on top is set. Cool for 15
minutes. Serve in dessert dishes, spooning sauce
from bottom of pan over each serving. Top with
ice cream or whipped cream and fresh raspberries,
if desired. Makes 9 servings.

## Fabulous Fig Bars

16 ounces Blue Ribbon Orchard Choice or
Sun-Maid Mission or Calimyrna Figs
1 cup packed brown sugar
1 large egg
½ cup chopped walnuts
1½ cups all-purpose flour
1/3 cup sugar
½ teaspoon baking soda
¼ cup rum or orange juice
1¼ cups old-fashioned oats
2 tablespoons hot water
½ cup butter, softened
*Rum Glaze, recipe follows*

Heat oven to 350° F. Coat 13 x 9-inch baking pan with cooking spray. Remove stems from figs and coarsely chop. Combine figs, walnuts, sugar, rum and hot water; set aside. Beat together butter and sugar until creamy. Add egg and mix until smooth. Stir in flour and baking soda; blend in oats to make a soft dough. Reserve 1 cup dough. With floured fingertips, press thin layer of remaining dough in bottom of prepared pan. Firmly pat fig mixture over dough. Drop reserved dough by teaspoonfuls over top, allowing fig mixture to show between drops. Bake 30 minutes or until golden brown. Cool completely in pan. Drizzle with rum glaze. Makes 36 bars.

Rum Glaze: Stir together ½ cup powdered sugar and 3-4 teaspoons rum or orange juice until smooth.

### Fruited Fig Dressing

½ cup lemon or limejuice
2 tablespoons walnut oil
6 California figs, stems removed
Dash salt
3 tablespoons fruit-flavored vinegar

Combine all ingredients in blender or food processor and blend smooth. Serve over mixed fruit, toss with assorted greens or drizzle over gilled chicken or tuna atop assorted greens. Makes about 2/3 cup.

### *White Chocolate-Fig Pie*

1½ cups (8 ounces) California figs, stems removed
2 eggs
1 package (12 ounces) white chocolate or confection, melted
1 (8-inch) graham cracker or chocolate crumb crust
2/3 cup half-and-half

Finely chop figs by hand or in food processor. Add melted chocolate, half-and-half and eggs, and process until smooth, or beat well. Turn into crust. Bake in preheated 350° F oven until knife inserted off-center comes out clean, about 30 to 35 minutes. Let cool completely. Refrigerate. Makes 1 (8-inch) pie, 12 servings.

### *Figgy Spread*

1 package (12 ounces) light or nonfat cream cheese *or* ricotta
¼ cup walnuts
1 teaspoon grated lemon peel, optional
1½ cups (8 ounces) California figs, stems removed
1 teaspoon cinnamon

Combine all ingredients in blender or food processor and blend until figs are coarsely chopped. Cover and refrigerate. Makes about 2 cups.

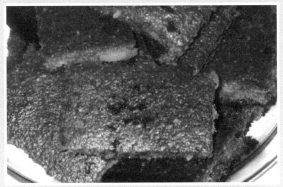
*Fresh Fig Cake*

### California Baked Apples with Walnuts and Figs

Two small baking apples
¼ teaspoon cinnamon
1 large dried California fig, finely chopped
¼ oz. California walnuts, finely chopped
¼ cup orange juice
½ teaspoon grated lemon zest

Preheat oven to 350°F. Core apples and pare one third of the way down. In small bowl, combine fig, 1 tablespoon of the orange juice, the walnuts, lemon zest and cinnamon. Using small spoon, stuff center and cover tops of apples with fig mixture. Arrange in small shallow baking dish and pour remaining orange juice over apples. Bake until tender, 45 minutes-1 hour, basting occasionally with orange juice.

### Fresh Fig Cake

3 cups cake flour
1 cup cream shortening
3 tsp baking powder
2 cups brown sugar
¼ tsp salt
Mix in 4 beaten eggs

1 tsp each cinnamon, nutmeg
Add 2 cups chopped raisins
½ tsp cloves together 3 times
½ lb figs, finely chopped

Directions: Add dry ingredients and one cup of water alternately, beating well. Pour into greased loaf pan. Bake at 350° F about two hours. Stirring frequently, until the consistency of marmalade. Add citrus fruit juice after you have removed from stove. Cool thoroughly before using.

### Chocolate Fig Pecan Bars

2 cups all-purpose flour
¾ cup chopped pecans
¾ cup sugar, divided
2/3 cup semisweet chocolate pieces
10 tablespoons butter or margarine, softened
3 large eggs
8 ounces Blue Ribbon Orchard Choice or Sun-Maid Mission or Calimyrna Fig, stemmed and chopped
¾ cup light corn syrup
1 teaspoon vanilla extract

Heat oven to 350° F. Stir together flour and ¼ cup sugar. Add butter. With pastry blender or 2 knives, cut butter into dry ingredients until mixture resembles coarse crumbs. (Mixture will be dry.) Press in bottom of lightly greased 12 x 9-inch baking pan. Bake for 15 minutes or until edges begin to brown. Sprinkle figs, pecans and chocolate pieces over crust. Lightly beat eggs, gradually beat in remaining ½ cup sugar, corn syrup and vanilla until blended. Pour over crust. Return to oven for 20 to 30 minutes or until filling is firm around edges and slightly soft at center. Cool on wire rack. Makes 32 bars.

## Baked Figs

10 fresh, ripe medium-sized figs, stemmed
2 tablespoons melted butter
1¾ ounces (50g) almond paste
1 ounce (30g) powdered sugar
10 sheets phyllo

Score the top third of each fig. Roll the almond paste into 10 equal balls. Press 1 piece onto the bottom of each fig. Cut each phyllo sheet into quarters. Stack four of these quarter pieces, staggering the corners. Brush the top sheet with melted butter and place a fig on the center of the stack. Wrap the sheets around the fig, making a beggar's purse. Brush the outside with melted butter. Repeat with remaining figs and phyllo. Bake the figs in a 300°F (150°C) oven until the figs are soft and the phyllo is golden brown, about 30 minutes. Dust with powdered sugar. *Serving Suggestion: serve with fresh raspberries.*

## Fig Date Parfaits

6 fresh figs
¼ cup raspberries
½ cup pecans, soaked
2 dates, pitted
1/3 cup raw maple syrup
2 tablespoons date soak water

Blend dates, soak water, and raspberries until smooth and set aside. Blend nuts and maple syrup until smooth, adding water if necessary. Cut figs into quarters, leaving bottom intact, and split open. Spoon nut crème into middle of open fig. Drizzle raspberry sauce on top. Garnish with fresh mint leaves or shredded coconut. Serves 2-3.

## Chewy Fig Granola Bars

½ cup *each* firmly packed brown sugar, salad oil and honey
3 cups rolled oats
1 cup crisp cereal
½ cup *each* wheat germ, flaked coconut and finely chopped almonds
¼ cup *each* sesame seeds and sunflower seeds
1 cup finely chopped California Dried Figs

In a small saucepan, combine brown sugar, oil and honey. Bring to boil over medium heat; simmer about two minutes. Preheat oven to 350° F. In a large mixing bowl, combine all remaining ingredients, except figs, stirring with a spoon or with mixer dough hook. Stir in sugar mixture until well blended. Add figs. Press mixture firmly into an ungreased 9 x 13-inch baking pan. Bake 20-25 minutes until toasty brown. Cool. Cut into narrow bars. Makes about 24 bars.

## Fig Trail Cookies

1½ cups whole wheat flour
¼ cup *each* honey and molasses
¾ cups all-purpose flour or oat flour
1 tablespoon finely grated orange peel
½ cup brown sugar, firmly packed
1 teaspoon vanilla
¼ cup wheat germ
1 cup orange juice
1 teaspoon *each* baking powder and cinnamon
1 cup chopped California Dried Figs
¾ cup golden raisins
2 eggs or 6 tablespoons egg substitute
½ cup chopped walnuts
1/3 cup melted margarine

Combine flours, sugar, wheat germ, baking powder and cinnamon. In smaller bowl, blend eggs, margarine, honey, molasses, orange peel, vanilla and orange juice with wire whip. Add liquid to dry ingredients, whip until smooth. Add figs, raisins, and walnuts. Spread in a greased 9 x 13-inch baking pan. Bake in a 350°F oven 35 minutes, until it tests done. Makes about 24 bars.

### Yam Bake a La Orange

2 large (1 lb. each) yams, boiled, peeled and sliced ¼ inch thick
¼ cup walnut pieces
¼ cup melted margarine
2 oranges, peeled and sliced
2 tablespoons honey
¾ cup California Dried Figs, sliced crosswise into fourths
1 teaspoon grated orange peel

Arrange yam slices, oranges and figs in an 8" round baking pan. Sprinkle with walnuts. Combine melted margarine, honey and orange peel. Pour over all. Cover with foil; bake in a 350° F oven for 30 minutes, until bubbly. Makes 6 servings

### Fig Aloha Cookies

1/3 cup butter or margarine
1 (8 ounce) can crushed pineapple, drained
½ cup sugar
1 egg
¼ cup chopped macadamia nuts or walnuts
1½ cups sifted flour
¼ teaspoon baking soda
½ cup chopped California dried figs

¼ teaspoon salt
Glaze: : 1 cup powdered sugar
2 tablespoons milk
Flaked coconut

In large bowl, beat butter, sugar and egg until fluffy. Combine flour, soda and salt; beat into butter-sugar mixture alternately with pineapple. Stir in nuts and figs. Drop by teaspoon on greased cookie sheet. Bake at 350° F for 10 to 12 minutes. While warm, dip cookies into glaze of powdered sugar and milk, then in coconut. Makes about 3-dozen.

### Figs in Port

*Try the fragrant figs over your favorite premium vanilla ice cream, or just pour a little heavy cream over a bowlful.*

1½ to 2 cups California figs, halved, stems removed
½ cup port
½ vanilla bean, split

Combine figs, port and vanilla bean in small saucepan. Cover and simmer until figs are very soft, about 30 minutes. Remove vanilla bean. Serve warm or chilled, with whipped cream or vanilla ice cream. *Note:* Add a tablespoon of lemon juice, if desired, and serve figs with roast pork. Makes about 4 servings.

1½ cups (8 ounces) California figs
1 round (9-inch) refrigerated pastry
or (8-inch) graham cracker or shortbread crust
1 cup orange juice
3 eggs

Combine figs and juice in blender or food processor until puréed. Add eggs and blend. Line a 9-inch tart pan or pie plate with pastry. Pour in fig mixture. Bake in preheated 375°F oven until a knife inserted off-center comes out clean, about 30 minutes. Let cool. Refrigerate. Makes 1 (8 or 9-inch) pie, 10 servings.

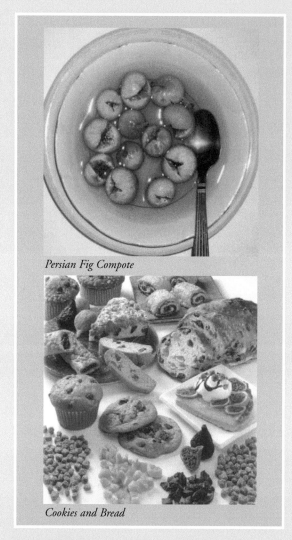

*Persian Fig Compote*

*Cookies and Bread*

### *Spiced Fig Compote*

1 (6-inch) strip orange peel
4 whole cloves
2 cups orange juice
1 cup Blue Ribbon Orchard Choice or
Sun-Maid Calimyrna Figs
½ cup sugar
2 cinnamon sticks
2 whole allspice
2 cardamom seeds, broken

In saucepan, combine orange peel, orange juice, sugar, cinnamon sticks, allspice, cardamom seeds and cloves. Bring to boil; simmer 5 minutes. Add figs; simmer, covered, 20 minutes. Serve warm or chilled. Store in refrigerator. Makes 8 servings. Or for a sweeter dish, prepare with Persian Baby Figs

### *Fig Pur*
*Use the purée as a jam, a filling for cookies or tarts, as an ice cream or fruit topping, as a drink sweetener or in your favorite barbecue sauce, salad dressing or glaze.*

### *Orange Fig Tart*

*Need a fancy dessert—fast? Here's the answer—only 4 ingredients but the result tastes like a fancy French pastry. The filling's consistency will remind you of pecan pie. California figs supply all the sweetness and orange is the perfect flavor partner.*

1 ½ cups (8 ounces) California figs
1 teaspoon vanilla
1/3 cup fruit juice (orange, lemon, lime, pineapple, cranberry or any blend) or water
½ to 1 teaspoon cinnamon
½ teaspoon nutmeg

Combine in blender or food processor and mix until puréed. Cover and refrigerate. Makes about 2 cups.

### White Chocolate-Fig Pie
*Make just two stops in the supermarket—the baking aisle for California figs and the crumb crust already in a pie pan, the dairy case for the eggs and half-and-half. Then spend less than 5 minutes with your food processor and.*

1½ cups (8 ounces) California figs, stems removed
2/3 cup half and half
2 eggs
1 package (12 ounces) white chocolate or confection, melted
1 (8-inch) graham cracker or chocolate crumb crust

Finely chop figs by hand or in food processor. Add melted chocolate, half-and-half and eggs, and process until smooth, or beat well. Turn into crust. Bake in preheated 350°F oven until knife inserted off-center comes out clean, about 30 minutes. Let cool completely. Refrigerate. Makes 1 (8-inch) pie, 12 servings.

## BREAKFAST FOODS AND BREADS

### Figgy Spread
*Here's the perfect way to add sweetness, flavor and fiber to a portable breakfast. Use the spread on toast, English muffins, scones or bagels. For a quick snack*

*or dessert, slather it on vanilla wafers, plain cookies or fresh apple or pear slices.*

1 package (12 ounces) light or nonfat cream cheese or ricotta
¼ cup walnuts
1 teaspoon grated lemon peel, optional
1½ cups (8 ounces) California figs, stems removed
1 teaspoon cinnamon

Combine all ingredients in blender or food processor and blend until figs are coarsely chopped. Cover and refrigerate. Makes about 2 cups.

### Fig and Walnut Pancakes
*No pancake house specialty can rival these hearty breakfast or brunch specials. Top with syrup if you need to, but they have plenty of flavor and substance to stand alone.*

1 cup California figs, coarsely chopped
½ teaspoon salt
½ cup coarsely chopped walnuts
2 eggs
1 cup all-purpose flour
1½ cups milk
1 tablespoon baking powder
1 tablespoon oil
1 teaspoon cinnamon
1 teaspoon vanilla
½ teaspoon nutmeg

In large mixing bowl stir together figs, nuts and dry ingredients. In separate bowl beat together eggs, milk, oil and vanilla. Add liquid mixture to dry ingredients and stir to blend. Pour about 1/3 cup batter for each pancake onto hot lightly greased griddle. Bake until bubbles on top break and batter is set at edges. Turn to brown other side. Serve hot. Makes about 12 (5-inch) cakes.

### Sweet Barley Porridge

4 cups barley, soaked
2 cups fig soak water
1 cup figs, soaked
2 teaspoons coriander

Blend ingredients to desired consistency. Add in extra figs just before stopping blender to provide chunks of fruit in this wonderful porridge. Serves 4-6.

### Grandma's Live Oatmeal Porridge

1 cup hulled oat groats, soaked
3 figs, soaked

Blend ingredients. In a pot, heat the porridge to 115°F or when hot to finger and serve.

### Amaranth Porridge

1 cup amaranth, sprouted
¼ cup figs, soaked
½ cup fig soak water
½ ripe banana

Blend all the ingredients until smooth. In a pot, warm to 115°F or until hot to the touch.

### Three Grain Muffins

1 cup each all-bran cereal, rolled oats and boiling water
1 cup California Dried Figs
1½ cups whole wheat flour
½ cup melted margarine or unsaturated oil (such as soy or corn)
1 cup unbleached or bread flour

(or ½ cup rye or millet flour and ½ cup unbleached)
2 eggs or 6 tablespoons egg substitute
1 cup buttermilk
1 teaspoon baking soda
½ cup each molasses and honey
1 teaspoon baking powder
1 teaspoon vanilla

In a medium bowl, combine bran cereal, oats and boiling water. Add melted margarine, eggs, buttermilk, molasses, honey, vanilla, and figs. In a large bowl, blend whole wheat and unbleached flours, soda and powder. Add liquid ingredients, mix lightly, just until blended. Spoon into greased muffin tins (do not use muffin papers, they will stick). Bake in a 400°F oven for 20 to 25 minutes. Makes 2 to 2½ dozen muffins.

### Sweet Sacred Challah

5 cups buckwheat, sprouted
2 cups figs, soaked and chopped
8 tablespoons flaxseed, ground

Separate dough into three equally sized strands and roll each in the ground flaxseed. Braid the three strands into one loaf. Dehydrate at 115 F for 10-12 hours, rather than bake.

**Read More About Figs in Your Garden
and Kitchen**

Berolzheimer, Ruth, Editor. *Culinary Arts Institute Encyclopedia Cookbook*, Perigee, 1988.

Cowin, Dana and Judith Hill, Editors. *Food and Wine 2000: An Entire Year's Recipes from America's Favorite Food Magazine.* American Express, 2000.

*Pasta & Italian*, Parragon Publishing, 2003
Staib, Walter et al. *City Tavern Cookbook: 200 Years of Classic Recipes from America's First Gourmet Restaurant*, Running Press, 1999.

Kessel, Janet, Fletcher et al. *California* (Williams-Sonoma New American Cooking). Time Life, 2000.

Printed in the United States
by Baker & Taylor Publisher Services